Short-Latency Auditory Evoked Potentials

SHORT-LATENCY AUDITORY EVOKED POTENTIALS
Fundamental Bases and Clinical Applications

THEODORE J. GLATTKE, PH.D.
Professor of Speech and Hearing Sciences
University of Arizona, Tucson

5341 Industrial Oaks Boulevard
Austin, Texas 78735

Printed in the United States of America

Library of Congress Cataloging in Publication Data
Glattke, Theodore J.
    Short-latency auditory evoked potentials.
    (Fundamentals of communication science series)
    Includes index.
    1. Electrocochleography. 2. Auditory evoked response.
I. Title. II. Series. DNLM: Evoked potentials, Auditory.
WV270G549s
RF294.5.E43G56   1983   617.8'82   83-1252
ISBN 0-936104-86-4 (previously 0-8391-1715-9)

5341 Industrial Oaks Boulevard
Austin, Texas 78735

10 9 8 7 6 5 4 3 2   85 86 87 88 89 90

CONTENTS

PREFACE

to Fundamentals of Communication Science

The publication of **Fundamentals of Communication Science** is undertaken with several purposes in mind. A primary objective is to produce a series of short, carefully prepared, scientifically sound, and clearly written introductory-level books concerning speech, hearing, and language. Each book is intended to address theoretical issues and/or empirical data which experts agree are the fundamental ideas and relations that define a particular area of knowledge. Each book is intended for a number of different courses taught in one or more departments in most colleges and universities.

Above all, we hope to contribute a series of useful and interesting books that will introduce undergraduate students to nationally known scholars who normally write original articles and evaluative reviews oriented toward other professionals and graduate students.

Constantine Trahiotis, Ph.D.
Charles E. Speaks, Ph.D.
Series Editors

PREFACE

This book is the outgrowth of the Course Notes that have accompanied several short courses I have taught during the past three years. Those courses were designed to provide the beginning user of cochleography and auditory brainstem response audiometry with a foundation on which to establish test procedures and interpretive guidelines. So it is with this book. The material contained here should help prepare the student or new practitioner to start the process of obtaining and evaluating recordings in a competent manner.

The scope of the book has been limited to cochleographic and brainstem response measures because of the tremendous popularity of those two procedures. The other types of auditory evoked potentials have not been treated, and the reader who is interested in them should consult any of the several reviews cited throughout the text.

Thanks are due to many individuals who helped in the efforts to gather and organize this material. Alfred C. Coats provided excellent criticism of the first rough version of the Course Notes. The students in the courses, with their questions and comments, have helped to determine both the scope and the level at which information has been presented. Constantine Trahiotis exercised great patience in waiting for the final manuscript, which was some two years in the making, and examined an earlier draft with an eye for clarity, accuracy, and relevance. It is a pleasure to acknowledge the contributions of all of these persons.

Most of all, I would like to acknowledge the support of my family during the times that this project kept me tucked away at the typewriter (later, word processor) or otherwise distracted me. My wife, Jean, carefully reviewed several sections from the viewpoint of a speech-language pathologist who often is confronted with ABR evaluation reports that are filled with jargon. She helped me to clarify several key points, and I am grateful for her assistance and persistence.

I hope that the reader will find the information contained herein to be pertinent, accurate, and helpful.

Ted Glattke

*This work is dedicated to
the late F. Mark Rafaty, M.D.
physician, teacher, and dear friend*

Short-Latency Auditory Evoked Potentials

1

INTRODUCTION

Auditory evoked potentials are of interest because they provide information about how the ear functions and how the brain responds to sound. These small changing voltages accompany many of the events that occur in the inner ear, auditory nerve, and central nervous system. Abnormalities of these responses may help to detect and locate disorders of the ear or nervous system. Until the mid-1960s, they were accessible only to experimenters who placed invasive recording electrodes in or near the tissue that generated the responses. Since that time, advances in the development of small flexible computers and sensitive amplifying systems have enabled clinicians and researchers to detect these minute responses from the surface of the body and to isolate them from irrelevant background electric activity. As a consequence, the study of auditory evoked potentials has become commonplace in the practice of audiology, neurology, otology, and related disciplines.

This book is about several types or classes of auditory evoked potentials and is organized around discussions of the origins of the responses, the principles and methods by which they are recorded, and the clinical findings that have been reported in the literature. It is convenient to classify the responses obtained from the auditory system on the basis of both their probable sites of origin and their latencies, or time intervals between stimulus arrival and response development. These

1

are summarized in Table 1.1. Responses classified by latency are designated as early-latency, middle-latency, and slow or late responses. While the cochlear and auditory nerve responses are in the early-latency range, they normally are designated according to their sites of origin. Within the early-latency time domain there may be found the auditory brainstem response (ABR), the frequency-following response (FFR), and a slow scalp-negative wave that appears about 10 msec after the stimulus arrives at the ear (SN-10). The middle-latency responses occur in the period between 10 and 100 msec after arrival of the stimulus at the ear, and the late responses appear in the 50 to 500 msec range.

Historical reviews of the various classes of responses may be found in Reneau and Hnatiow (1975), Simmons and Glattke (1975), Davis (1976), Gibson (1978), Glattke (1978), and Fria (1980). That information will not be repeated here. This book is designed to answer such questions as "How may the responses be recorded?"; "Why should this or that procedure be followed?"; and "How should the results be interpreted?", and focuses on three types of responses that have been of increasing interest and value to clinicians in the past few years. These are: (1) responses from the cochlea; (2) the *whole nerve action potential* (AP) of the auditory nerve; and (3) *the auditory brainstem response* (ABR). In order to begin studying these responses, it is necessary to review basic applied physiology of the auditory system.

OVERVIEW OF THE EAR

Traditionally, the ear is considered to be composed of four parts defined according to their structure and function. As illustrated in Figure 1.1,

Table 1.1   Classification of auditory evoked potentials by response latency and site of origin

Response classification	Latency range (msec)	Probable origin
Cochlear		
Cochlear microphonic (CM)	~0	Cochlear hair cells
Summating potential (SP)	~0	Cochlear hair cells
Auditory nerve responses		
Whole nerve AP	1.5–4.5	Auditory nerve
Early-latency responses		
Auditory brain stem response (ABR)	1.5–8	Auditory nerve and brainstem
Frequency-following response (FFR)	7–10	Cochlea, auditory nerve and brainstem
Scalp-negative wave (SN-10)	9–12	Unknown
Middle-latency responses	10–100	"Primary" auditory cortex
Late responses	50–500	"Primary" and "association" cortex

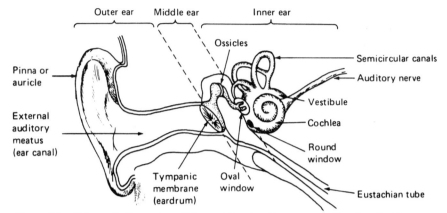

Figure 1.1.   Schematic illustration of the peripheral auditory system. Reprinted with permission from Glattke (1980).

these divisions are (1) the *outer ear*, consisting of the auricle or pinna, and the external meatus; (2) the *middle ear*, including the tympanic membrane, ossicles, middle ear muscles, the Eustachian tube, and the middle ear cavity; (3) the *inner ear*, with its vestibular and cochlear portions; and (4) the *auditory nervous system*, which begins with the *auditory nerve* (cranial nerve VIII) leading from the inner ear to the brainstem. Each of these parts of the ear plays an important role in the processing of auditory stimuli, and so each influences the characteristics of the evoked responses obtained by auditory stimulation.

The outer ear is an acoustical device. Its role in humans is to help to capture sounds and to provide some protection for the tympanic membrane. It is well known that humans are able to detect sounds ranging in frequency from about 20 Hz to 20,000 Hz, but that our hearing is most sensitive in the middle range of frequencies between about 1,000 and 4,000 Hz. The outer ear sets the stage for our sensitivity to mid-frequency sounds by acting as an acoustical resonator in the process of conducting sound down to the tympanic membrane. Primarily because of the length of the external meatus (about 2.5 cm), the outer ear offers a boost in the *sound pressure level* (SPL) of sounds in the region of 2,500 to 3,500 Hz. Perhaps the most important aspect of the outer ear that must be considered in a clinical evoked-potential setting is its patency. An external meatus that is occluded due to cerumen or other debris or to collapse of its soft cartilaginous outer portion simply will not conduct sound to the tympanic membrane. This suggests that the first step in obtaining auditory evoked potentials would involve examination of the external meatus and a means of checking to insure that the pressure of the stimulus earphone does not cause the meatus to collapse. One should be especially alert to the possibility of collapse of the meatus in neonates and also in geriatric patients.

The middle ear operates as a combined acoustical and mechanical device. Sound arriving at the tympanic membrane sets it into motion. The three auditory ossicles (malleus, incus, and stapes) transmit that motion to the oval window of the inner ear and hence, to the fluid that surrounds the sensory apparatus within the inner ear. The moving parts of the middle ear system constitute a transformer mechanism that improves the efficiency of the transfer of energy between the air of the external meatus and the fluid within the inner ear. The major element of this transformer is the ratio of the area of the tympanic membrane to the area of the stapes footplate that fits into the oval window. The slight pressure that is effective in moving the tympanic membrane is increased at the stapes approximately 17 times due to the area-ratio mechanism. In addition to this transformer action provided by the tympanic membrane and ossicles, the middle ear system operates as a filter. The middle ear cavity is like a small drum, and the air trapped within the cavity makes the tympanic membrane very stiff. This stiffness prevents the ear from responding very efficiently to low-frequency sounds, and so helps to "tune" the ear to the preferred midfrequency range. The normal ventilation of the middle ear cavity is afforded by the Eustachian tube, which opens during swallowing to allow air to pass between the pharynx and middle ear cavity. If the Eustachian tube remains closed for an appreciable period, the air pressure within the middle ear cavity will decrease relative to the ambient pressure. This will change the stiffness characteristic of the tympanic membrane and make the ear's response to low-frequency sounds even poorer than normal. Chronic obstruction of the Eustachian tube leads to the accumulation of fluid in the middle ear cavity. From an acoustical point of view, the fluid reduces the volume of air in the cavity and increases the stiffness of the tympanic membrane. If enough fluid accumulates to contact the membrane itself, the membrane motion becomes very limited and significant hearing loss will result. A middle ear cavity that contains fluid will produce a hearing loss that is greatest in the low-frequency range. Some types of middle ear (conductive) hearing loss may extend into the high-frequency range, however. The individual with a longstanding history of middle ear disorders often may be compromised further. The maximum hearing loss due to disruption of the middle ear system can extend to about 60 dB, or about half the range of intensity produced by most audiometers.

Since many of the measures used to help interpret evoked potentials are sensitive to the amount of hearing loss a patient may have, it follows from the foregoing that an evaluation of the integrity of the middle ear apparatus should be a part of clinical evoked-potential studies. This evaluation would seem to be especially important for very young children who may have undetected middle ear disorders and for head-trauma patients who may have experienced fracture of the temporal bone. In addition to the possibility of damage to the inner ear, the head-trauma patients may have blood or other fluid in the middle ear or external meatus, and may have a tear in the tympanic membrane. Those factors could cause very misleading changes in the responses.

The inner ear, the first part of the auditory system to produce electric responses of clinical interest, functions to convert mechanical activity into nerve excitation. The patterns of motion of the stapes are communicated to the fluid of the inner ear, and the motion of the fluid causes vibration of the *organ of Corti* within the cochlea. The organ of Corti consists of a pair of membranes with specialized receptor cells sandwiched between them. When the membranes are set into motion, resulting mechanical stimulation of the hair (receptor) cells causes the necessary excitation of the nerve fibers attached to those cells. There are about 15,000 hair cells in the inner ear and a part of the action of the cochlea is to provide for "selective" excitation of them. The excitation patterns of the hair cells are the result of the cochlea's mechanical analysis of the incoming sounds. High-frequency sounds result in stimulation of receptor cells located near the basal coil of the cochlea, while low-frequency sounds are most effective in stimulating cells in the cochlea's upper turns. The mechanical analysis also disperses the excitation of the hair cells in time. The cells that receive maximal stimulation from the high frequencies respond very quickly after the arrival of the stimulus at the inner ear. Cells responding to lower frequencies receive their stimulation 3 or more msec after those driven by high-frequency stimulation. This analysis scheme is related intimately to the pattern of excitation of nerve fibers in the auditory nerve, and it will be discussed more completely in Chapter 3.

When the cochlear encoding process is disrupted, the patient is said to have a *sensorineural* hearing loss. There are many different causes of inner ear disorders that lead to hearing loss, but they can be grouped into those that change the mechanical action of the inner ear, those that cause disruption of the metabolism of the inner ear, or those that result in the loss of hair cells (and nerve fibers) of the inner ear. The hearing loss due to inner ear disorders may be uniform across all frequencies, may be confined to the low frequencies, or, more commonly, may involve the high-frequency region exclusively. Since the normal cochlea establishes complex tuning and timing patterns for hair cell and nerve fiber stimulation, it follows that many of the characteristics of the auditory evoked potentials will be quite sensitive to the status of the cochlea. The interpretation of auditory evoked potentials from a neurological standpoint must be couched in terms of the logical effects of possible cochlear disorders.

The principal parts of the auditory nervous system are illustrated in Figure 1.2. The first element, the auditory nerve, enters the brainstem at the junction of the medulla and pons. The auditory nerve ends at the *cochlear nucleus* (CN), which consists of two major divisions: dorsal and ventral. Neurons arising from the dorsal CN tend to project to midbrain structures after crossing the brainstem near the floor of the fourth ventricle. Neurons from the ventral CN carry information into the *superior olivary complex* (SOC) on both sides of the brainstem. The SOC is the "lowest" auditory center to receive significant input from both ears and apparently provides the first analysis that permits us to locate sounds in space. Neurons that exit from the SOC travel in a fiber tract that forms the *lateral lemniscus* (LL) and passes to the *inferior colliculi* (IC). The *commissure* of the IC provides a pathway for neurons to cross the brain

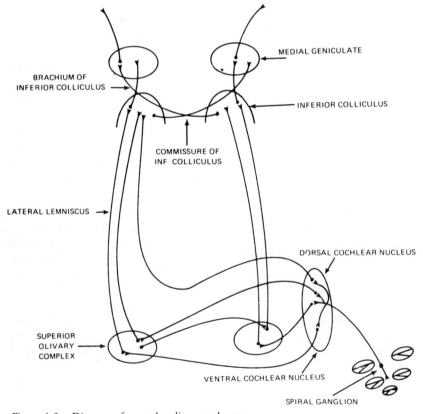

Figure 1.2.   Diagram of central auditory pathways.

at the midbrain level, and the *brachium* of the IC carries neurons to the *medial geniculate bodies* (MGB). Auditory system neurons radiate diffusely to the cortex from the MGB region.

Although the auditory nuclei of the brainstem, midbrain, and thalamus are often described as "way stations" that simply pass information along to the cortex for decoding, the facts seem to point to those structures as sophisticated analyzers, involved with the recoding of information about the complexity of the stimuli. For example, neurons in the CN may provide selective responses only to the onset of sounds, while elements in the SOC respond preferentially as the result of combinations of stimuli at the two ears. In the IC, one encounters selective responses to changes in ongoing sounds, such as may occur in speech. The brainstem and midbrain nuclei certainly are not homogeneous, and probably do not make uniform contributions to the evoked responses obtained in a clinical setting.

Disorders of the auditory nervous system include tumors or other space-occupying lesions, degenerative diseases, infection, or the consequences of malformation or trauma. Often, they may escape detection with a conventional hearing threshold test and will be demonstrated only through evaluations involving sophisticated listening tasks or other diagnostic procedures. It is in this area that the evaluation of the various classes of auditory evoked potentials offers great promise. The ABR, when interpreted in the context of the status of the peripheral auditory mechanism, has exquisite sensitivity to a variety of disorders of the central nervous system. When ABR measures are combined with cochlear and auditory nerve response analysis, the precision with which space-occupying lesions can be located is often as good as that provided by modern x-ray techniques. Chapters 2 and 3 continue this review of basic auditory physiology, with an emphasis on the origins of the cochlear, auditory nerve, and brainstem responses.

SUMMARY

The auditory system may be divided into four distinct parts on the basis of anatomic and functional criteria. The outer and middle ear portions tend to shape the overall response of the ear so that midfrequency sounds are emphasized. Disruption of the outer and middle ear systems will affect the results of evoked potential studies if that disruption causes a significant hearing loss. The analysis of sound performed by the inner ear is a major determinant of the pattern of electrical responses obtained from the auditory nerve and brainstem structures. Hearing loss due to inner ear disorders may be expected to influence auditory evoked responses in a manner consistent with what is known about how the inner ear operates. Inner ear disorders may be expected to result in changes in many of the features of the responses, including their thresholds, latencies, and general waveforms. Neurological disorders may also produce changes in the characteristics of the responses, and an important task for the clinician who would use auditory evoked potentials lies in the separation of effects due to hearing loss from those due to neurological disorders. These relationships will be described further in subsequent chapters.

2

COCHLEAR ELECTRICAL POTENTIALS

Electrical potentials generated within the cochlea are grouped into two classes: *resting potentials* (extracellular and intracellular), present when no known stimulus has been delivered to the ear, and *stimulus-dependent potentials* that become apparent when the ear is stimulated by sound (Dallos, 1973).

The illustration in Figure 2.1 provides a cross-sectional view of a single cochlear turn and summarizes the findings of Lawrence, Nuttal, and Clapper (1974) regarding the distribution of cochlear resting potentials. When a small electrode enters the fluid-filled space of the scala media, a steady direct current (dc) voltage having a magnitude of about + 80 millivolts (mv) relative to the rest of the body is encountered. First described by von Bekesy (1950), this steady voltage reflects the chemical composition of the endolymph and depends on the integrity of the stria vascularis for its maintenance. This extracellular potential is known as the *endolymphatic potential*. Electrodes that penetrate single cells within the organ of Corti detect voltages of about − 70 mv relative to the body surface (Tasaki, Davis, and Eldredge, 1954). The intracellular potential is found within the supporting cells of the organ of Corti and the cochlear receptor or hair cells. Interestingly, the fluid spaces enclosed within the

9

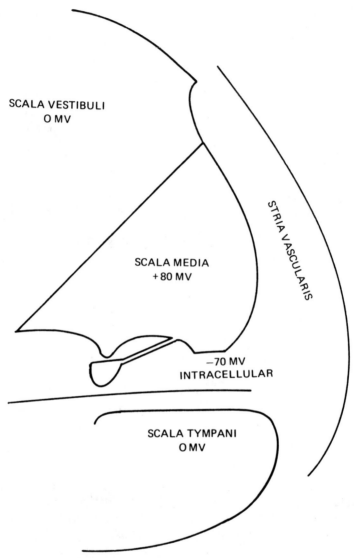

Figure 2.1.   Distribution of dc resting potentials within the cochlea. Redrawn from Lawrence, Nuttal, and Clapper (1974).

organ of Corti reveal no positive potential relative to perilymph, suggesting that the tectorial membrane provides an insulating barrier between the organ of Corti and the endolymph.

The stimulus-dependent potentials are the *cochlear microphonic* (CM) and the *summating potential* (SP).

The microphonic is an alternating current (ac) potential that appears to follow the waveform of the auditory stimulus with good fidelity. More precisely, Dallos (1973) argues convincingly that the CM is a manifestation of the motion patterns of hair cells, and is dominated by the outer hair cells in the normal ear. Several of the characteristics of the CM recorded from an electrode placed on the round window of a normal laboratory animal are illustrated in Figure 2.2. Figure 2.2A is a photographic record of the CM in response to the presentation of a 1,000 Hz sinusoidal stimulus having a duration of 12 msec. The lower tracing was obtained by reversing the phase of the tonal stimulus. Note that the upper tracing begins with a negative-positive-negative deflection pattern, while the lower tracing is inverted relative to the upper. In Figure 2.2B, the stimulus frequency was changed to 2,000 Hz. The two tracings illustrate the CM associated with a change in the stimulus sound pressure level (SPL) of 6 dB. That 50% reduction in pressure is reflected precisely in the change in amplitude of the CM.

The CM appears with essentially no time delay between the arrival of the stimulus at the cochlea and CM onset. In a normal recording situation where an earphone is used to generate the response, the CM has a latency that reflects the travel time of the stimulus through the outer and middle ear apparatus, about 130 microseconds (μsec). This feature of the CM helps to fix its origin in the cochlea, as opposed to the nerve fibers leading from the cochlea. The neural response generally is delayed by more than 1 msec after the arrival of the stimulus at the ear.

Because the CM is intimately related to the condition of the cochlear hair cells, recordings of the CM have been proposed as a clinical tool.

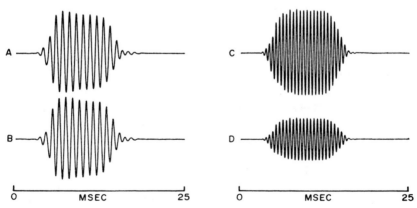

Figure 2.2.   Cochlear microphonic recordings for various stimulus conditions: (A) 1,000 Hz tone burst; (B) 1,000 Hz tone burst with phase reversed; (C) 2,000 Hz tone burst; (D) 2,000 Hz tone burst with SPL reduced by 6 dB.

The appeal of the CM for clinical purposes lies in the speculation that loss of hair cells in specific regions along the length of the organ of Corti might be manifested by selective loss of the CM for various test frequencies. As mentioned in Chapter 1, high-frequency signals elicit mechanical activity that is restricted to the lower or basal region of the cochlea, and low-frequency signals cause mechanical disturbances that travel relatively further toward the cochlear apex. Tasaki, Davis, and Legouix (1952) introduced a CM recording technique that has been used with great care by Dallos (1973) to demonstrate that the CM recorded from restricted regions of the cochlea mirrors the general pattern of mechanical activity within the cochlea. The specialized "differential electrode" recording technique allows one to measure the CM generated in the vicinity of a pair of electrodes placed above and below the scala media in one turn of the cochlea by cancelling CM potentials that originate more than a few millimeters from the recording site. This powerful technique allows the experimenter to determine precisely which region is contributing to the CM, but it cannot be used clinically because placement of the electrodes requires surgery that poses serious risk to the patient.

Clinical recordings of the CM are made with an electrode placed near the cochlea, for example, on the inner wall of the middle ear cavity, on the floor of the ear canal, or on the earlobe. The utility of CM recordings is very limited, due to two factors related to this placement. The first is that any distant electrode site causes a reduction in maximum CM voltage from the millivolt range down to less than 1 μv (microvolt). The fractional-microvolt magnitude of the CM can be obtained only with relatively intense auditory stimuli. Intense stimuli composed of low frequencies are known to cause mechanical excitation along a great length of the cochlea, from the base toward the apex. Because of the extent of stimulation, it is not possible to determine which region of the cochlea is contributing to the CM. The second factor compromising the interpretation of the CM is that it is dominated by hair cells that are closest to the electrode site (Simmons and Beatty, 1962).

Thus the remote sites used for clinical recordings make speculation regarding specific site(s) of origin of the CM tenuous, at best. The major contribution of CM recordings to differential diagnosis at present seems to be limited to fixing site of lesion in a gross way (Beagley and Gibson, 1978). For example, if the CM may be detected in the *absence* of any responses from the auditory nerve, one suspects a disorder involving the nerve rather than the cochlea. If neither CM nor auditory nerve responses are detected, the general site of lesion is placed within the cochlea.

Sometimes, the CM may obscure other types of desired electric potentials when relatively long duration tone bursts are used to elicit responses. Two procedures may be used to reduce or eliminate the CM from recordings intended to emphasize neural components. The first involves *filtering* the physiologic recording and selecting an auditory stimulus that has a frequency range outside of the range of the filter. Since the CM follows the waveform of the stimulus (approximately) it will be eliminated by the action of the filter. The general effects of filtering electrical signals corresponding with physiologic activity will be described in Chapter 4. The second method of eliminating the CM from the recording makes use of the fact that the CM follows the phase of the stimulus. An averaging system is configured to sample the CM and other response components for a number of repetitions of the stimulus at a fixed starting phase. The stimulus phase is then reversed (as in Figure 2.2B), and the computer samples the responses to an equal number of repetitions of the stimulus. When the electrical responses from the normal and the phase-reversed stimuli are summed in the computer memory, the CM voltage adds to zero, and electric potentials *that do not follow the stimulus waveform* emerge from the CM or other sources of contamination. This result is illustrated in Figure 2.3. The upper tracing was obtained from repeated samples of a tone burst. Note that the CM is not symmetric about the baseline, by comparing the A and B amplitudes. The CM is nearly eliminated in the lower tracing and what emerges is a small baseline shift that has a duration equal to the period of stimulation. This small baseline shift is the dc summating potential.

Like the CM, the SP is strongly influenced by the status of the cochlear hair cells, and it appears to be sensitive to disorders that involve the status of the hair cells (Coats, 1981). In the normal ear, the SP detected by electrodes placed at sites used for clinical studies accompanies the CM and appears as a very small (0.05 to 0.5 μv) *negative* shift in the baseline of the recording. Like the CM, the SP has essentially no latency between the arrival of the stimulus at the ear and the onset of the response. In addition, the SP and CM persist for the duration of the stimulus without significant adaptation, or loss of amplitude. Unlike the CM, the SP does not appear to mimic the stimulus waveform, but has a constant polarity. (It is a dc voltage.) Clinically, the appearance of abnormally large SPs suggests a disorder involving the cochlea.

SUMMARY

Two classes of cochlear electric potentials, the CM and the SP, may be detected with electrodes normally used for clinical evaluation of humans.

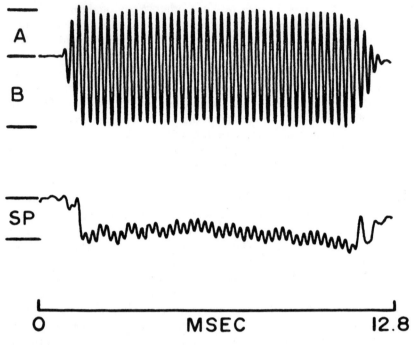

Figure 2.3.   Example of cancellation of the CM and the appearance of the SP. The SP is a small baseline shift that occurs with the CM. Note the difference between the baseline and peak measures *A* and *B* in the upper tracing. The distance between the baseline and *B* is greater and is due to the presence of the SP. After cancellation of the CM, the SP may be seen clearly in the lower tracing.

Their characteristics are linked closely to the condition of the hair cells. The usefulness of the CM and SP to point to specific sites of lesions along the length of the organ of Corti is very restricted, however. The CM and SP can be distinguished from electric potentials of neural origin on the basis of their latency, waveform, and persistence throughout the duration of the stimulus. The latency to the onset of the CM and SP is vanishingly small. The CM waveform mimics the pattern of displacement of the hair cells and bears a strong resemblance to the waveform of the auditory stimulus. The SP waveform, by contrast, appears as a small dc shift that has a duration equivalent to that of the stimulus. The persistence of both the CM and SP marks these potentials as end-organ, possibly generator potentials, rather than electric events of neural origin.

3

ELECTRICAL ACTIVITY
IN THE AUDITORY
NERVE AND BRAINSTEM

The whole nerve AP of the auditory nerve and the ABR are complex electric responses that result from the discharges of a great number of neurons. Both types of responses are so closely related to cochlear function that the clinical practice of Electrocochleography includes consideration of both the AP and ABR in some laboratories. Because of the intimate relationship between cochlear events and the subsequent short-latency neural responses, this chapter reviews cochlear mechanical activity very briefly before turning to specific considerations of the AP and ABR.

Energy arrives at the cochlea through a piston-like motion of the stapes. The stapes follows the waveform of the auditory stimulus with modifications imposed by the acoustic and mechanical properties of the outer and middle ear systems, which, as noted previously, behave like a broadly tuned filter to provide the best coupling between the inner ear and airborne sound in the frequency region between 1,000 Hz and approximately 4,000 Hz.

The motion of the stapes displaces the fluid within the cochlea, and the scala media reacts to the fluid motion with a series of undulations that appear to start at the basal end, near the stapes, and travel toward the apex. Grossly, the motion pattern developed by the scala media appears something like the pattern that would develop for a rope that was fixed at one end and then shaken in a rhythmic pattern by someone holding the free end. There is an important difference between the motion patterns of the scala media and those of the simple rope, however. In the case of the rope, the undulations would travel down the entire length until they reached the fixed end, while the disturbance that travels along the scala media covers a distance determined by the *frequency of the stimulus.*

The moment-to-moment displacement patterns of the scala media are complex, reflecting the mechanical characteristics of the organ of Corti. Estimates of the extent to which the motion pattern travels down the length of the scala media can be illustrated as in Figure 3.1. The schematic illustrations of Figure 3.1 represent the *envelopes* of the displacement patterns, rather than showing the fine details of those patterns. Low-frequency stimuli, below about 100 Hz, result in disturbances that travel the full length of the cochlea and require about 5 msec to complete the trip from base to apex. Midrange frequencies of approximately 1,000 to 2,000 Hz elicit disturbances that travel about half the length of the cochlea, reaching their final destination in 1 to 2 msec. High-frequency stimuli have mechanical activity patterns that are confined to the basal region of the cochlea and complete their travel within 100 to 200 μsec after the onset of stapes motion. The patterns of activity illustrated in Figure 3.1 reflect not only the fact that the travelling waves terminate at well-defined positions within the cochlea, but also that the mechanical

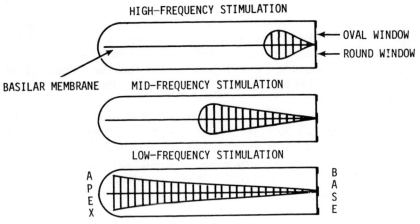

Figure 3.1.   Schematic illustration of the cochlea (uncoiled) and travelling wave envelopes for various stimulus frequencies.

disturbance grows to some maximum value before ending its travel. Note that the mechanical disturbance is reduced sharply beyond the point of maximum displacement.

These activity patterns reflect the tuning determined by the physical characteristics of the basilar membrane. The membrane is about 0.05 mm wide at the basal end of the cochlea and about 0.5 mm wide near the cochlear apex. The change in width of the basilar membrane corresponds with a gradation in *stiffness*, and the basal region is about 100 times stiffer than the apex. When other physical attributes (mass, friction) are held constant, a relatively stiff mechanical system will have a preferential response for rapid motion patterns, or those caused by high-frequency stimuli. A system with a relatively little stiffness, such as the cochlear apex, will be *unable to respond rapidly* to high-frequency stimuli and will have a preferential response to low-frequency stimuli. This mechanical tuning is the basis for the ear's ability to separate complex stimuli into their component frequencies. Each stimulus arriving at the inner ear will result in travelling wave patterns that mirror the frequencies contained in the stimulus, and the cochlea will, to the limits of its resolving power, develop individual travelling waves for each of the component frequencies in a complex stimulus. The magnitude of the displacement patterns is in the sub-angstrom (diameter of a simple molecule) range for stimuli near the threshold of hearing, and it grows in direct proportion to the sound pressure level (SPL) of the stimulus. In the case of complex stimuli, the magnitudes of several travelling waves that might be present simultaneously are presumed to reflect the magnitudes of each of the frequencies in the stimulus. The moment-to-moment displacement patterns in the cochlea also reflect the stimulus frequencies that elicit those patterns. A high-frequency stimulus will drive the portion of the basilar membrane that responds to it at a high rate of vibration. A very low-frequency stimulus will drive the *entire* basilar membrane at a corresponding lower rate.

The cochlear displacement patterns ultimately result in excitation of the hair cells by mechanisms that are not understood completely. It is generally believed that the cilia projecting from the top of the hair cells are displaced either by fluid trapped beneath the tectorial membrane or by virtue of their contact with the membrane itself. Motion of the cilia results in a change in the electrochemical properties of the hair cells, and that reaction results in excitation of the nerve fibers that innervate the cells.

The afferent, or sensory, nerve supply leading from the cochlea is organized according to the scheme illustrated in Figure 3.2 (Spoendlin, 1973). The vast majority of the nerve fibers group together in very short

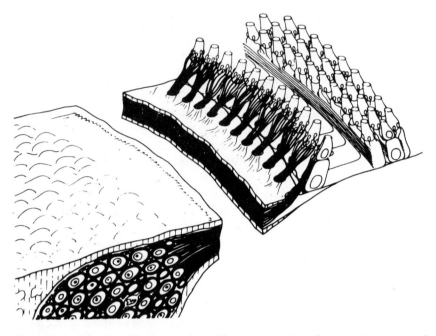

Figure 3.2.   Schematic illustration of the afferent innervation of the cochlea. Reprinted with permission from Spoendlin (1973).

bundles that concentrate on the inner hair cells. About 20 fibers attach to each inner hair cell. Because of this precise point-to-point innervation, the discharge patterns of individual auditory nerve fibers reveal several characteristics of the analysis of stimuli by the cochlea. By studying the characteristics of individual neurons, we can begin to answer the question of which nerve fibers in the auditory nerve contribute to the whole nerve action potential.

GENERATION OF THE AP

The electrical activity of single auditory nerve fibers may be recorded only with very small microelectrodes that detect events within individual fibers. The response from an individual fiber consists of a very brief electric pulse, or "spike." This spike-like discharge is the result of a rapid reversible change in the electrical state of the fiber.

The clinical measures of auditory nerve responses are based on recordings taken with relatively large electrodes placed near the cochlea. The large electrodes cannot detect the individual spikes produced by individual fibers unless special invasive recording procedures are used

(Kiang, Moxon, and Kahn, 1976). Rather, the large electrodes detect voltages that represent the complex sum of the small discharges from active nerve fibers. Examples of the waveforms detected in both types of recording situations are illustrated in Figure 3.3.

Our understanding of the link between discharge patterns of single neurons and the whole nerve AP response has been increased by the research of Kiang and his co-workers (Kiang, 1965; Kiang and Moxon, 1974; Kiang, 1975; Antoli-Candela and Kiang, 1978). The following discussion is based on their findings.

The first property of auditory nerve fibers that is relevant to our question is their *tuning.* The tuning may be demonstrated by stimulating the ear with pure tones of different frequencies and determining the minimum SPL required for each of those tones to elicit a response from the nerve fiber. The resulting data, relating threshold SPL to different frequencies, is displayed as a *tuning curve.* Representative tuning curves for several individual nerve fibers are illustrated in schematic form in Figure 3.4. As the curves imply, the single fiber response is confined to a very narrow frequency range until the stimulus SPL is raised to a moderately intense level. The "best" or *characteristic frequency* (CF) of a nerve fiber is the stimulus frequency that requires the *least* SPL to elicit a response from the fiber. The CF of the fiber therefore corresponds to the location of the sharp tip of its tuning curve. The sharpness of the

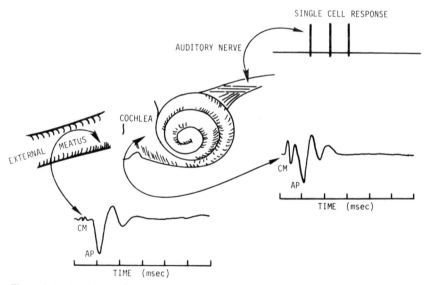

Figure 3.3.   Examples of the whole nerve AP responses obtained from the cochlear promontory and from the ear canal, and single neuron spike responses recorded from the auditory nerve. Modified with permission from Coats and Jerger (1979).

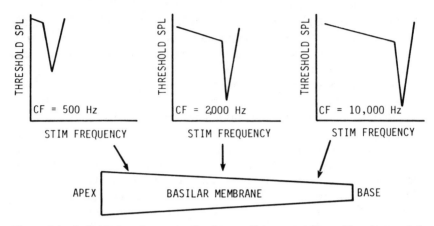

Figure 3.4.   Individual tuning curves for three auditory nerve fibers. The characteristic frequency (CF) of the neuron requires the minimum SPL to elicit a response. The region of the cochlea innervated by the neuron is related to the CF of that neuron.

tuning curves suggests great precision in the tuning for each fiber. Because of the precision of the fiber tuning and what is known about the innervation patterns of neurons, *a fiber's point of origin in the cochlea may be estimated on the basis of the CF.* A neuron having a high CF must originate in the basal region of the cochlea, and apical fibers have preferential responses for low stimulus frequencies.

The precise tuning occurs for low and moderate stimulus SPL. Single fiber tuning curves also reveal a lengthy "tail" extending into the low-frequency range for intense stimuli. This tail reflects the fact that the travelling wave that develops for low-frequency stimuli arises from the basal (high-frequency) end of the cochlea before making its way to the region where it results in the most efficient stimulation of receptor cells. The long tail on the tuning curve suggests that high-intensity stimuli of low frequency (e.g., 500 Hz) will cause nerve fiber excitation throughout the cochlea.

Stimuli that are most effective in eliciting the AP response must have an abrupt onset or *rise time* (Goldstein and Kiang, 1958), to provide the basis for *synchronous* discharges from a great number of neurons. Examples of whole nerve AP responses obtained from a laboratory animal for stimuli having various rise times are illustrated in Figure 3.5. Enhancement of the response with abbreviations of the onset of the stimulus is quite apparent. The problem posed by the use of clicks or brief tones, however, is that the *energy associated with those stimuli disperses throughout the audible spectrum.* This spread of energy leads to uncertainty as to which region of the cochlea is receiving maximal stimulation, and, therefore, which nerve fibers are contributing to the whole nerve AP.

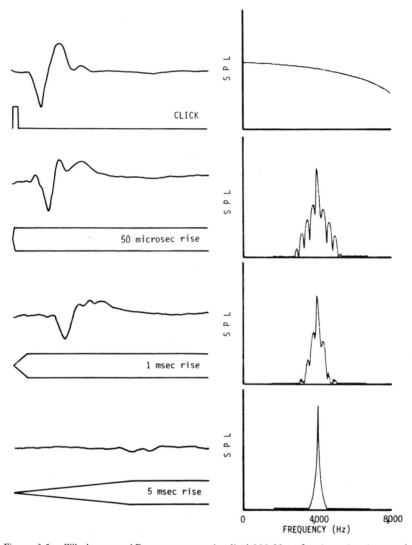

Figure 3.5.   Whole nerve AP responses to stimuli (4,000 Hz) of various rise times and to click stimuli. The amplitude spectrum of each stimulus is illustrated to the right of each example.

Part of the uncertainty can be resolved if the *time delay* associated with the travelling wave in the cochlea is considered. Very brief time delays are encountered for the travelling waves due to high-frequency stimulation, and progressively longer delays correspond with low frequencies. The time delay between the onset of a stimulus and the first response from a single auditory neuron is determined by that neuron's position in the cochlea and can be predicted by the CF of the fiber. Single neurons having CFs in the low-frequency range *cannot* respond to a click stimulus with a time delay, or latency, of only 1 or 2 msec because they are located relatively far from the base of the cochlea. For moderate and high stimulus intensities, the whole nerve AP response begins to develop within 1 to 2 msec after the stimulus arrives at the ear. Because very brief response latencies imply that the basal, or high-frequency, fibers are contributing to the response, one can conclude that the AP response is *dominated by neurons that innervate the basal region of the cochlea in the normal ear for moderate- or high-intensity stimuli.* These very brief response latencies always imply that the response is dominated by the basal region of the cochlea, regardless of the frequency of the auditory stimulus.

Direct evidence supporting these concepts has been provided by the simultaneous recording of activity of single neurons and the AP response. An examination of the relationship between the neuron CF, the latency of the neuron response, and the peaks of the AP response has led to the construction of "neurograms" for click stimuli (Kiang, 1975; Antoli-Candela and Kiang, 1978). In Figure 3.6 one of these neurograms illustrates the discharge patterns for 50 single neurons in response to a click stimulus of moderate intensity. The discharge pattern for a single neuron is illustrated by a horizontal line that has one or more peaks as it progresses from left to right in the figure. The peaks represent increases in neuron discharge rate, and they occur at latencies indicated by the horizontal axis (0 to 4 msec). The receding position of each of

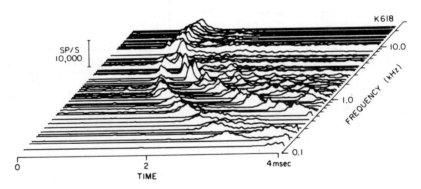

Figure 3.6. Neurogram display of spike activity for 50 individual neurons in a single animal. The stimulus was a brief click presented at a peak SPL of 100 dB. Reprinted with permission from N.Y.S. Kiang, "Stimulus representation in the discharge patterns of auditory neurons." In D. B. Tower (ed.), *The Nervous System, Vol 3: Human Communication and Its Disorders.* New York: Raven Press, 1975.

the lines that represent activity of a single neuron is fixed by the CF of the neuron and indicated along the frequency axis. Neurons having CFs in the lower-frequency range (cochlear apex) are located in the front of the display, and neurons with high-frequency CFs (base) are represented by tracings toward the rear of the figure.

Examination of the neurogram reveals that the response peaks having the briefest latency are located toward the rear of the illustration and therefore are attributed to neurons that innervate the basal region of the cochlea. Neurons innervating the basal region of the cochlea also tend to discharge during a single brief time "window." Neurons tuned to middle and low frequencies respond with multiple, progressively delayed bursts of spikes. The intervals between the peaks on the neurogram grow larger as the CF of the fibers progress to lower frequencies. The intervals may be predicted by the period of the CF of the neuron. For example, the interval between response peaks for a neuron with a 1,000 Hz CF will be 1 msec. The interval will be approximately 2 msec for a neuron with a CF of 500 Hz. These repeated discharges are evidence for a sustained mechanical "ringing" activity along the basilar membrane. They are of more than passing interest, because they extend into the time period normally associated with the ABR and may make a contribution to that class of evoked response.

Changes in stimulus SPL result in alterations of the AP response and those alterations also present a problem for interpretation of the responses. Figure 3.7 illustrates whole nerve AP responses obtained for click stimuli from a human subject with normal hearing sensitivity. The response makes its appearance at threshold as a slight undulation in the baseline of the recording. As the SPL of the stimulus is increased the response grows slowly with each increment until the stimulus is 50 to 60 dB above threshold. Further increases in the level of the stimulus are accompanied by a relatively rapid growth of the response and a change in the response waveform from a single peak to a series of succinct negative peaks. In addition to the changes in response amplitude and shape, the normal AP response latency also changes with increases in the stimulus SPL.

What causes these latency and amplitude changes? Evans (1975) and Ozdamar and Dallos (1976) have offered the following reasonable explanations. In general, a click stimulus has a very broad spectrum. When it is presented to the ear at near-threshold intensities, the filtering action of the outer and middle ear apparatus (as well as the natural preferred response of the earphone) results in an emphasis of the mid-frequency region. This energy concentration elicits an AP response with a moderately long latency (2 to 4 msec). As the click stimulus SPL is increased two events occur. First, progressively more high-frequency energy be-

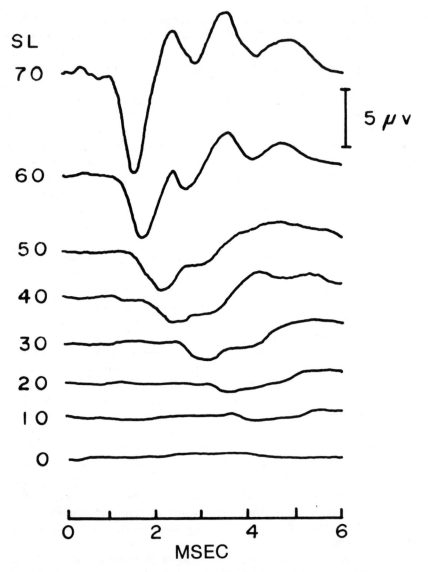

Figure 3.7. Examples of whole nerve AP responses obtained for a normal listener. The stimulus sensation level (SL) is noted beside each tracing.

comes effective in eliciting responses from the cochlea and auditory nerve. Second, the energy concentrated in the midfrequency region becomes effective in driving neurons that innervate the basal region of the cochlea. The more basal contributions are reflected in (1) a decreased response latency and (2) a narrower time "window" during which the initial portion of the response may appear. The growth of the response represents the progressive addition of neurons to the response and the fact that the added neurons discharge in very close registration with each other. The close registration provides for a summed response that, in addition, to having a brief duration, has a greater amplitude than if the fibers' spike responses were distributed over a longer time period.

In summary, the whole-nerve AP is the result of the discharges of a great number of single auditory neurons. The AP is detectable only when a sufficient number of neurons discharge in close registration. This close registration is made possible by the use of an auditory stimulus that is very brief or has an abrupt onset. The requirement for an abrupt onset results in an uncertainty as to which region of the cochlea may be contributing to a response. For example, ears with significant damage to the basal region of the cochlea would generate AP responses with prolonged latencies, because neurons usually capable of responding after the briefest latency would be eliminated by the damage. Prolonged responses may also be associated with other types of problems, however, including simple conductive hearing loss or disorders involving the auditory nerve. Hence, interpretation of the AP response without complete information as to the status of the ear that has been tested is tenuous, at best. Techniques that have been introduced to improve the audiometric precision of the AP response measurements will be reviewed in Chapter. 6.

GENERATION OF THE ABR

The ABR offers many of the same problems of interpretation posed by the AP. Examples of ABRs obtained for click stimuli are illustrated in Figure 3.8. The near-threshold response is a small baseline shift that occurs with a latency of about 8 msec after the arrival of the stimulus. As the intensity of the stimulus is increased, the response takes the form of multiple succinct peaks.

Soon after the ABR found its way into clinical applications, a number of authors suggested that the multiple response peaks could be associated with *sequential activation* of the auditory nerve, brainstem, and midbrain structures (Lev and Sohmer, 1972; Stockard, Stockard, and Sharbrough, 1977). Wave I was attributed to the auditory nerve. Wave II was identified with the cochlear nucleus. Wave III was linked to activity of the superior olivary complex, and waves IV and V were thought to be due to activity of the lemniscal pathways and inferior colliculi. An implication of this scheme is that lesions of the central nervous system could be

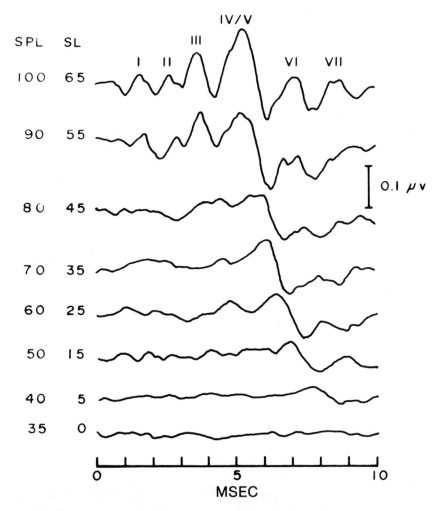

Figure 3.8.   Examples of the auditory brainstem response obtained for a normal listener. The stimulus SPL and sensation level are noted beside each tracing.

located with great precision by examining the response for the loss or modification of one or more of the response components.

More recent evidence suggests, however, that while wave I does appear to be dominated by electrical activity due to the auditory nerve, the concept of individual generators for the later response components is not appropriate. This more recent evidence comes both from studies that compared electrical activity *within* the brainstem and midbrain to the surface-recorded ABR and from those studies that involved the introduction of controlled lesions. The response-comparison studies in-

SURFACE   ABR

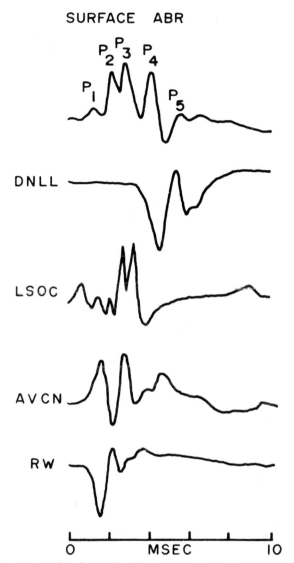

Figure 3.9.   Examples of surface and indwelling recordings of responses of cat auditory system to click stimuli. RW = round window; AVCN = anterio-ventral cochlear nucleus; LSOC = lateral superior olivary complex; DNLL = dorsal nucleus of the lateral lemniscus. The stimulus SPL was approximately 57 dB. From Runge (1980).

clude those of Achor and Starr (1980a) and Runge (1980), who examined responses in cat. Both studies demonstrated that the major structures of the brainstem responded to click stimuli with *sustained* electric activity, and so it was not possible to demonstrate that a single site can be specified as the sole generator for a specific response peak.

Examples of Runge's (1980) data are illustrated in Figure 3.9. The top tracing is the ABR obtained from surface electrodes in cat. It is characterized by multiple peaks (P_1-P_5), and the largest of those, P_4, is thought to be analogous to wave V in humans. The bottom tracing is an example of a simultaneous response obtained from the auditory nerve via an electrode placed on the round window of the cochlea. The other responses were obtained from the cochlear nucleus, superior olivary complex and lateral lemniscus, respectively. The coincidence between the surface response and two or more of the responses obtained from the intracranial electrodes is obvious in the illustration. Similar observations throughout brainstem and thalamic regions have been made in human subjects by Hashimoto et al. (1981). Moller and his colleagues have also investigated human subjects using intracranial electrodes, and have suggested that the first two components of the human ABR are both influenced strongly by the auditory nerve response (Moller, Jannetta, and Moller, 1981, 1982; Moller and Jannetta, 1982). They also speculated that there was probably no midbrain (inferior colliculus) contribution to wave V in humans. According to their findings, the generators for the first five waves in humans are located in the lower brainstem; this coincides with the theories of Kevanishvili (1980, 1981).

The lesion studies of Achor and Starr (1980b) also suggest that there are multiple contributors to the various components of the response. Among their general findings, they noted that a single lesion could affect several of the response peaks in cat. They also observed that lesions in different locations could all affect a single response peak. Finally, they reported that when an animal was allowed to recover from the surgery necessary to place a lesion certain portions of the aberrant response recovered, even though the primary lesion remained intact.

SUMMARY

The whole nerve action potential response is due to the complex electrical summation of the discharge of a great number of individual nerve fibers. The overall pattern of the response can be explained well by a consideration of the timing of the discharges from the neurons that contribute to it, and the timing of those discharges is related to the mechanical analysis performed by the cochlea. In general, high-frequency or high-intensity (regardless of intended frequency) stimuli will elicit a whole nerve response dominated by neurons that arise from the basal region of the cochlea in the normal ear. This knowledge allows us to begin to interpret abnormal auditory nerve responses in terms of damage to particular regions of the inner ear or portions of the auditory nerve.

There is general agreement that wave I as detected in the ABR corresponds with the major peak of the whole nerve response. The auditory nerve also appears to contribute to wave II and perhaps later response components. The latency characteristics of the normal ABR are thought to reflect cochlear processing in the manner of the auditory nerve response, and so the ABR obtained for high-intensity stimulation is considered to be dominated by neurons that respond preferentially to high-frequency stimulation.

The central nervous system sources for the individual peaks of the ABR have not been identified with certainty. Proposed sources for wave V include structure extending from the low brainstem to the midbrain (inferior colliculus). In spite of lack of definitive information regarding the sources of the ABR, abnormalities of the response latency and waveform often correlate well with the presence of a disorder of the central nervous system. More detailed information regarding normal and clinical findings will be reviewed in Chapters 7 and 8.

One important group of factors that influences the outcome of clinical evoked potential studies falls under the heading of methodology. This will be the subject of Chapter 4, which reviews the principles underlying the stimulation and recording of responses in order to provide a basis for understanding how modifications of recording or stimulus techniques can influence the characteristics of the response.

4

METHODOLOGICAL CONSIDERATIONS IN STUDIES OF HUMAN EVOKED POTENTIALS

An examiner's ability to detect auditory evoked potentials and the characteristics of those responses are influenced strongly by stimulation and recording techniques. Special techniques are needed to extract the desired response from irrelevant electrical "noise." The noise includes: (1) electrical activity produced within the body of the person from whom the recordings are obtained; (2) interference from electrical radiation; (3) artifacts produced by the generation of the auditory stimuli that elicit the response; and (4) electrical signals present in the recording apparatus. In most cases, the desired response is very small and is concealed by the background electroencephalogram (EEG) activity and other electrical noise produced by the patient. Detecting the response requires the use of special apparatus such as that illustrated in Figure 4.1. The most important part of the apparatus is a computer system that stores samples of the patient's electric signals (EEG activity) that are coincident with the presentation of the auditory stimuli. However, the first step toward

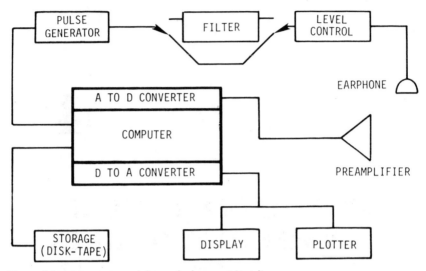

Figure 4.1.   Apparatus used for evoked potential studies.

reducing the unwanted noise involves the use of special EEG pream-plifiers called *differential preamplifiers*.

PREAMPLIFIERS

Differential preamplifiers capable of detecting cochlear and neurogenic electric activity have the following characteristics:

1. They have very low internal electrical noise.
2. They have a broad frequency response range (dc through 10,000 Hz).
3. They allow the examiner to select a frequency range that is most appropriate for the desired response.
4. They allow detection of the patient's electrical signals at *three* electrode locations.

A preamplifier is illustrated in schematic form in Figure 4.2. The three electrodes placed on a patient typically are identified as the *active*, *reference*, and *ground* electrodes.[1] The active electrode, placed on the

---

[1] These conventional terms are a bit misleading. Traditionally, an "active" electrode was placed near or within the tissue that was responsible for generating the response. The "reference" electrode was placed at a site where little or no relevant activity could be detected. The "ground" electrode was coupled to a true earth ground point. The "active" and "reference" sites for typical ABR and other evoked potential studies are both elec-trically active. That is, the response may be detected from either the "active" or "reference" site. Due to electrical safety requirements, modern recording systems do not use a true earth ground connection.

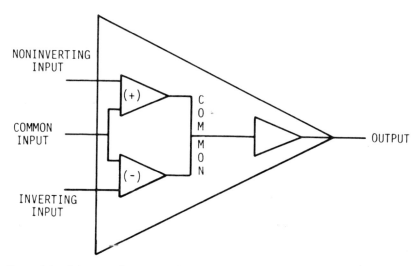

Figure 4 ?   Schematic illustration of a differential preamplifier.

vertex of the skull, is led to the *noninverting* input of the preamplifier. The reference electrode is led to the *inverting* preamplifier input. The ground electrode is led to a *common* input and is placed on the forehead.[2] There are at least three amplifier circuits inside the unit. The noninverting input signal is led to a circuit that amplifies the signal present between the active and ground electrodes. An identical amplifier stage accommodates the signal between the reference and ground electrodes, and it *reverses* the phase or electrical polarity of that signal. The outputs of the two initial stages are added together on a common electrical pathway before being led to subsequent stages within the amplifier. The effect of the addition of the noninverted and inverted signals on the common pathway is the *elimination* of voltages that were present with identical characteristics at the active and reference electrode sites. *Only the difference between the signals at the active and reference sites is led to the subsequent amplifier stages.* This cancellation of electrical signals that are identical at the electrode sites aids in the detection of the desired evoked response because much of the unwanted noise in the test environment is present at both the active and reference sites.

---

[2] Unfortunately, there is no standard connection scheme for the active and reference electrodes. When the vertex electrode is led to the noninverting preamplifier input, electrical signals that appear as positive voltages at the vertex will be seen as positive voltages at the preamplifier output. The opposite occurs when the vertex electrode is coupled to the inverting input of the preamplifier, and electrically negative signals detected at the vertex will be seen as positive voltages at the output. The majority of reports dealing with ABR studies display vertex-positive voltages in an upward direction, but several significant publications follow the opposite convention. Caution is required of the reader!

An example of the application of differential amplification is illustrated in Figure 4.3. The signal applied to the noninverting input consists of a small EEG voltage plus a large fluctuating voltage due to electrical radiation from nearby incandescent lights. The large sinusoidal voltage is radiated 60-Hz ac power supplied to the lights. The signal applied to the inverting input consists of the same 60-Hz noise and a small EEG voltage that is not identical to that present at the noninverting input. At the outputs of the first amplifier stages, the noninverted signal has the same phase as the input, but the inverted signal contains the large 60-Hz component as a mirror image of the upper tracing. When the non-inverted signal and the mirror image are added together the unwanted 60-Hz component is cancelled and the small differences between the EEG signals are passed through the amplifier system. As the example in Figure 4.3 illustrates, the unwanted noise that is cancelled by the preamplifier may be much larger than the intended signal. Therefore, the differential preamplifier provides a significant first step in reducing the unwanted noise, or improving the signal-to-noise ratio. The amount of discrepancy between unwanted noise and desired signal that can be accommodated by a differential preamplifier is specified as its *common-mode rejection ratio*, in dB. In a typical recording situation, the desired ABR often is only .01 to .001 of the ambient electrical noise, and the minimum common-mode rejection ratio required of the preamplifier is 60 dB (1:1000 voltage ratio).

Electrode Locations and Impedance   In an ideal recording situation, the noninverting and inverting inputs will be attached to electrodes that (1) detect equal amounts of noise, artifacts, and other unwanted

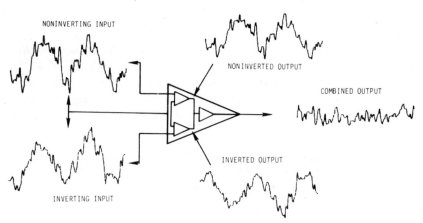

Figure 4.3.   Schematic illustration of noise cancellation effects of a differential preamplifier.

voltages *and* (2) detect the desired response in a manner that does not compromise its appearance at the output of the preamplifier.

The first ideal criterion listed above would be met if the active and reference electrodes were very close together, but under that circumstance the noise and the desired response would both appear very similar at the two electrode sites. The differential preamplifier would, therefore, reduce both the noise and the desired signal. If the electrodes were separated by a great distance, for example, head-to-toe, one could insure that the signal would be detected much differently at the two sites, but the unwanted noise may also be different at the two locations and would not be cancelled efficiently. A suitable approximation of the ideal condition typically is met with all recording electrodes on or near the head. An example of an ABR detected by a noninverting electrode on the vertex, an inverting electrode on the mastoid ipsilateral to the stimulated ear, and a common electrode on the forehead is illustrated in Figure 4.4. The ABR waveform detected at the noninverting site consists of a series of voltage fluctuations that includes a rather broad IV/V complex. The ABR detected at the mastoid also contains a relatively broad IV/V complex that does not coincide exactly with the complex detected at the vertex. Subtraction of the mastoid waveform from the vertex waveform produces the response illustrated on the right of the figure. The resulting wave V is a sharp voltage fluctuation located approximately in the middle of the IV/V complexes seen at the individual electrode sites. The positioning of the other response components results from similar combinations of the electrical events seen at the two electrode sites. An

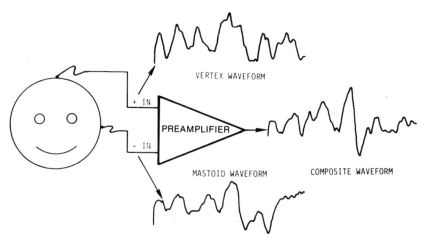

Figure 4.4.   Examples of the ABR detected at the vertex and mastoid sites, and the combination effects of the differential preamplifier. The common electrode was placed on the forehead and is not illustrated.

important implication of the example in Figure 4.4 is that *the choice of electrode sites will have a significant effect on the form, or morphology, of the response* (cf. Picton et al., 1974; Parker, 1981). Modification of the response can include changes in the number of components, the amplitudes of the peaks and the apparent latencies of the individual waves.

A major factor that determines whether the active and reference electrodes detect the same amount of unwanted noise is how well they are coupled to the skin of the patient. The electrodes must be mechanically secure to prevent movement artifacts. Even small amounts of electrode movement will result in the generation of electrical signals that may overdrive the sensitive preamplifier system and prevent detection of the desired cochlear or neural signals. The electrodes must also have excellent electrical contact with the skin so that they do not present a significant barrier to the detection of the response. The continuity between each electrode and the skin is checked by measuring electrode *impedance*, by passing a very small electric current between the individual electrodes and the indifferent electrode. A suitable meter provides a display of the impedance of each of the electrode pairs (Durrant and Phillips, 1979). The amount of electrical noise present at the input to the preamplifier system will be directly related to the amount of electrode impedance. Poor electrode connections will be reflected in high impedance values and will be accompanied by unsatisfactory noise levels. Good continuity is associated with impedance values in the 1,000- to 2,000-ohm range. A more subtle problem occurs when the active and reference electrode impedances are not matched: the electrode with the higher impedance will detect more noise than the electrode having the low impedance, and any differences between the noise levels present at the two electrode inputs will be amplified along with the desired signals.

Suitable electrode continuity first requires that the skin be cleaned to remove debris and oil. After cleansing, the electrode site is rubbed to remove superficial skin, and a special conductive paste is applied to the site. The paste is also applied to the electrode surface, and the electrode is pressed onto the prepared site.

The following application technique has proven to be very reliable for placement of the vertex electrode. The site is cleaned with a gauze sponge saturated with alcohol. An abrasive paste, such as Redux or Omniprep, is applied to the site and rubbed into the skin with a dry gauze sponge. The site is cleaned a second time with an alcohol sponge. A small amount of electrode paste, such as Grass EC-2, is applied to the site. The electrode surface receives a generous coating of electrode paste and the electrode is applied to the paste on the skin. A small cotton ball is coated on one side with additional paste and then pressed, paste side down, onto the recording electrode. No adhesive tape or other mechanical attachment is required at the vertex site when this paste-electrode-paste-cotton ball "sandwich" is used, although it is desirable to provide strain relief for the electrodes by taping their lead wires to the side of the head.

The forehead, earlobe, or mastoid sites do not require vigorous abrasion, and the examiner may prefer to use tape to cover the electrodes placed on those sites. If tape is used, the amount of electrode paste applied to the skin and electrode surface should be reduced so that it does not spread out beyond the edge of the electrode disk and prevent the tape from adhering to the skin. Common electrode materials are gold, silver, or tin disks attached to the preamplifier inputs by long flexible wires. It is a good practice to braid the wires together over much of their length to reduce further the effects of radiated or other electrical noise.

FILTERS

The filters included with EEG amplification systems also help to reduce the irrelevant background noise. The amount of noise passed by an amplifier system will be related directly to the total frequency range passed by the amplifier. If the noise is distributed randomly among all of the frequencies passed by the amplifier, the noise level will be reduced by an amount predicted exactly by the bandwidth of frequencies eliminated by the filters. Therefore, preamplifier filter settings are selected to eliminate electrical noise in a frequency range that is not important to the response.

Traditional EEG recordings that can be displayed on conventional strip-chart recorders consist of very low-frequency electrical activity. As a result, the late evoked potentials derived from those EEG signals can be recorded through amplifier systems that pass only those frequencies below about 20 Hz. The middle, early, and cochlear response require correspondingly greater frequency ranges. As a general rule, the filter setting should span the frequency range from the lowest frequency of interest to a value equal to *twice the highest frequency of interest*. The upper frequency limit for ABR and whole nerve AP studies typically is 3,000 Hz or greater. Failure to employ the appropriate minimum filter bandwidth may reduce the response amplitude and distort the apparent intervals among response peaks (Laukli and Mair, 1981). Further, if one uses extremely narrow filter settings, faulty electrodes that normally would be detected by the presence of unacceptable noise levels may not be discovered. Because no general agreement has been observed by individuals who have contributed to the literature on evoked potentials, the reader must be alert to procedural differences that may produce apparently conflicting findings.

COMPUTER-BASED SAMPLING

The computer system employed in evoked potential studies is very critical to the problem of noise reduction. The computer will control the timing of the stimulus presentations, the period over which the EEG or other electrical signals are sampled, and any computations that might be required after sampling has been completed. The most important computer-based function is the computation of an average of the EEG signals (or cochlear responses) that occur coincidentally with the presentation of repeated stimuli. The steps associated with averaging of evoked potentials are as follows:

1. A stimulus is initiated and routed to the earphone.
2. As soon as possible, the computer begins to sample the ongoing EEG signal as rapidly as is required to preserve the fidelity of that signal. The sampling is accomplished by an *analog-to-digital converter*, which captures the EEG voltage at some instant and expresses the magnitude of that voltage as some number. The number is then added to the contents of a designated location in the computer's memory. This procedure is repeated until the patient's electrical activity has been sampled for a sufficient time period, such as 10 msec after the onset of the stimulus. The individual sample captured in this manner may consist of 500 or more numbers, each representing the EEG voltage at a brief moment after the stimulus onset.
3. After a sample of 500 or so data points has been gathered and converted to numerals, the sample is added to the results of previous sampling in the computer memory on a point-by-point basis.
4. When all of the sampling is complete, the computer determines the *arithmetic mean* corresponding to each datum point by dividing the accumulated sum in each memory location by the number of samples gathered to obtain that sum.
5. This mean response then is displayed or plotted for analysis. If some form of digital storage is available, the plotting and subsequent measurement may be deferred until a more convenient time.

The individual memory locations where numerals representing the moment-to-moment changes in the EEG signal are stored are sometimes called computer *bins*. The amount of time required for the computer's analog-to-digital converter to capture, convert, and store a single data point is called the computer *dwell time* or bin width. The computer dwell time must be short enough to allow the computer to capture the fine details of the response. The dwell time determines the computer's sampling rate (not to be confused with stimulus repetition rate), and that sampling rate should be at least twice as high as the highest frequency passed by the preamplifier filters. Typically, the computer systems designed to capture ABRs have a sampling rate of 50 kHz, or about 15 times the usual 3,000 Hz upper filter setting.

Another important characteristic determined by the computer's architecture is the precision with which it can represent numbers. Numerals are stored in the computer memory in a binary format as strings of 1s and 0s called *bits*. The length of that string determines the range of numbers that the computer can accommodate without loss of data. The analog-to-digital converter must be able to express voltages as numbers that are compatible with the computer's requirements and that can span the range between the small ABR and its accompanying background noise. The range between typical background noise and the ABR is so great that the minimum length of the numbers from the analog-to-digital converter should be 12 bits in order to capture the small ABR. This allows the EEG and other voltages to be divided into 4,096 (2^{12}) steps, which is satisfactory for our purposes. (The error that results from using shorter number lengths (8 or 10 bits) is similar to the rounding error associated with small calculators that display only a few digits. The ABR is so small that it occupies the "least significant" part of the number, and can disappear with a rounding error.)

The computation of an average of the EEG activity associated with replications of the stimulus is necessary because the desired response remains concealed within the background EEG activity, even after the proper application of electrodes and the action of the preamplifier. The desired response appears following averaging of the data because it is present *consistently* in each of the samples obtained by the computer. By contrast, the unwanted noise that does not occur consistently develops an average value of zero or near-zero. The amount of noise reduction required is determined by the relative magnitudes of the desired response and the background noise. For example, a typical ABR has a maximum amplitude of about 0.1 to 0.5 μv. The ABR often is hidden in a background noise of 10 to 30 times the magnitude of the response. In order to detect the response, the background noise must be reduced by a factor of about 10 to 30. The amount of noise reduction that can be expected may be predicted by the total number of samples obtained before computation of the mean response. The noise reduction is equivalent to a factor equal to the square root of the total number of samples. The illustrations in Figure 4.5 provide examples of how the noise reduction proceeds with increments in sample size. Following the rule just

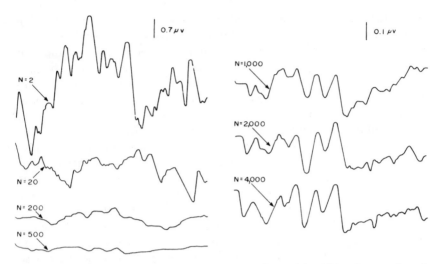

Figure 4.5.   Effects of increasing sample size on the form of the ABR. *N* = number of samples associated with each response. Note 7-fold increase of plotter sensitivity for the responses on the right.

stated, increasing the sample size by a factor of 10 will reduce the noise to a mean amplitude of about ⅓ the magnitude of individual samples. A 100-fold increase of the sample will result in a noise reduction to ¹⁄₁₀ the noise of an individual sample. Gathering 1,000 samples will reduce the noise to about ¹⁄₃₀ that found in an individual sample. As may be noted from Figure 4.5, a crude rendering of the ABR is visible after 200 samples have been taken, but clear definition of the response components is not apparent until about 1,000 samples are gathered. Increasing the sample size from 1,000 to 2,000 samples does not correspond with a significant enhancement of the response, because each time the sample size is doubled, the noise is reduced by only about 30%. The potential gain in response clarity associated with a very large number of samples, such as more than 2,000, usually is offset by the great amount of time required to obtain the additional samples. In contrast to the ABR, the middle and late evoked potentials require smaller sample sizes because of their favorable size relative to concurrent background noise.

DESCRIPTIONS OF TYPICAL STIMULI

Three types of stimuli are used to obtain the cochlear and early latency responses: acoustic clicks, tone pips, and tone bursts. The illustrations in Figure 4.6 provide examples of how these stimuli are produced and the general appearance of their waveforms.

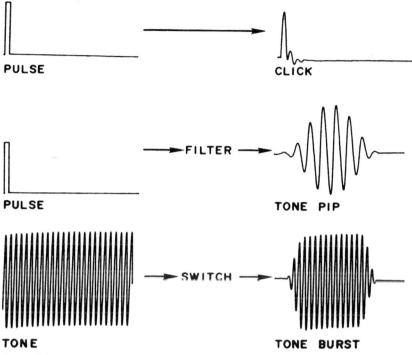

Figure 4.6.   Examples of waveforms of typical stimuli.

Clicks are produced by sending a brief electrical pulse to the earphone. It should be emphasized that the earphone does not respond to the pulse with a single brief displacement of its diaphragm. Rather, the earphone response will be a complex waveform consisting of several rapid cycles (Tobias and Jeffress, 1962). This "ringing" action is similar to that which occurs when a crystal glass is tapped lightly. The predominant frequency associated with the response of the earphone will be determined by its mechanical characteristics, the duration of the applied electrical pulse, and how the earphone is coupled to the listener's ear (Coats and Kidder, 1980). Changes in the spectrum of the click may be expected to result in change of the latency and other characteristics of the whole nerve AP response and the ABR. Since standards for the generation of the click stimuli are lacking, comparison of normative data among clinics and laboratories frequently is compromised by variations related to the type of earphone selected, the duration of the pulse, and other factors.

Frequently, reports will be encountered that describe the use of *rarefaction, condensation,* or *alternating* clicks. A rarefaction click is a stimulus that is produced by initially pulling the earphone diaphragm away from the tympanic membrane. A condensation click is produced by initially pushing the diaphragm toward the tympanic membrane, and alternating stimuli switch back and forth between the two initial modes of diaphragm displacement. The initial phase of the stimulus and the intensity of the stimulus interact in a complex way to produce changes in the latency of responses of auditory nerve fibers (Antoli-Candela and Kiang, 1978). Changes in the discharge patterns of auditory nerve fibers can be expected to contribute to changes in the AP and ABR potentials in a complicated manner. The lack of a standard technique is detrimental to the development of uniformly accepted response norms. The use of alternating clicks frequently is recommended as a way to eliminate the cochlear microphonic and "stimulus artifacts" from a mean record based on repeated sampling. If the CM or artifact are mirror images of each other as the stimulus is alternated, then this technique will be successful (see Figure 2.3). However, the response of conventional earphones to high stimulus levels (where the artifacts become troublesome) may not be perfectly symmetric when the electrical input is reversed. The rarefaction response may not be a mirror image of the condensation response, and the cancellation will be incomplete. The incomplete cancellation may result in serious distortion of the apparent AP or ABR response waveform. Individuals who wish to use the alternating-polarity stimulus technique would be wise first to demonstrate complete cancellation electronically before attempting to collect responses from patients. One way of accomplishing this is to present the alternating clicks to the subject accompanied by a masking noise sufficient to mask the response. The resulting mean should contain no neural response (AP or ABR), no evidence of the masking noise (since it would cancel during averaging), and no stimulus artifact (or cochlear microphonic). Brief latency voltages that do remain can be subtracted from the response obtained without masking in order to arrive at a less-distorted response waveform. If the stimulus artifact is so great as to "saturate" the preamplifier or computer, this cancellation technique will not be practical.

Tone pips are formed by leading an electrical pulse through a narrowband filter before passing it on to the transducer (Davis, Silverman, and McAulfie, 1951). The resulting waveform reflects the ringing action of the filter, and the stimuli are sometimes referred to as "filtered clicks." The principal frequency produced by the action of the filter will be the nominal center of the band of frequencies passed by that filter. If a frequency change is desired, one simply changes the center frequency of the filter band. If the relative width of the filter is held constant (e.g., ⅓ octave) then the pips produced in this manner will have exactly the same number of cycles, regardless of the center frequency. For example, the pips may have a pattern that rises to a maximum amplitude in three or four cycles and then decays in three or four cycles. When the center frequency is changed, the *time required for the filter ringing action also changes*. For example, if a filter is set to 500 Hz, it will ring for 12 to 16 msec. The same filter reset to 4,000 Hz will ring for only 1.5 to 2 msec to complete a six- to eight-cycle pattern. This means that there is an unavoidable interaction between the time over which a stimulus develops and the nominal frequency of the tone pip. That interaction may cloud the interpretation of responses to tone pips, including the measures of latency of the responses.

Tone bursts are generated by gating an ongoing electrical signal through an electronic switch or by some other modulation technique. The stimulus duration and frequency can be controlled independently. The stimulus rise time interacts with frequency in a complicated way. The higher frequencies can rise from zero to maximum amplitude very rapidly because of the brief duration of each of their cycles. Lower frequencies require correspondingly longer rise times. A very brief rise time causes the energy of the stimulus to spread to a band of frequencies on both sides of the intended signal. (See Figure 3.5.) Since the rise time, however specified, interacts with stimulus frequency and spectral dispersion, some uncertainty about point of stimulation in the cochlea accompanies the use of tone bursts and tone pips.

AMPLITUDE MEASURES

The amplitudes of stimuli used to elicit evoked responses are reported in various ways in the literature. Three common scales of measurement are (1) *sound pressure level* (sometimes noted as peak-equivalent SPL); (2) *sensation level* (SL); (3) *normal hearing level* (nHL). The SPL of a stimulus usually refers to the root-mean-square average pressure created by that sound in a conventional earphone calibration apparatus. The slow response of the metering equipment used to display SPL requires that the stimulus have a long duration. Clicks, tone pips, and other brief stimuli cannot be measured in a meaningful way using the conventional apparatus. The SPL of a brief stimulus is estimated by using a continuous signal having a frequency located at the principal frequency of the brief stimulus. This two-step procedure is illustrated in Figure 4.7. The calibration apparatus is arranged to include an oscilloscope capable of displaying the brief waveform of the voltage produced by the calibrating microphone. The amplitude of that voltage is noted, and then the brief signal is replaced by a continuous sinusoidal signal. The sinusoidal signal amplitude is adjusted until the microphone voltage output matches the peak value observed for the brief signal. The SPL of that sinusoidal is

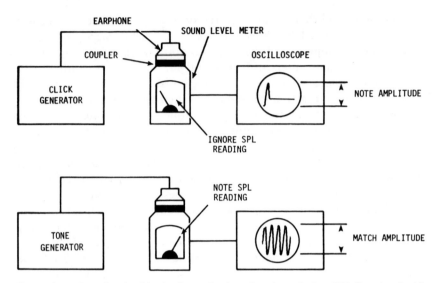

Figure 4.7.   Steps involved in the determination of peak-equivalent SPL. Reprinted with permission from Coats and Jerger (1979).

taken as the peak-equivalent SPL of the brief signal. Any amplitude expressed as N dB SPL is always referenced to a standard pressure of 0.0002 dyne/cm^2 (20 μPascals). (N dB = 20 log P_2/P_1, where P_2 is the pressure of the signal and P_1 is the reference pressure.) The click stimulus perceptual threshold typically is 30 to 35 dB peak-equivalent SPL for normal young adult listeners.

The SL scale was borrowed from psychoacoustics. When used correctly, the expression N dB SL refers to a stimulus that is N dB *above the patient's perceptual threshold for that stimulus*. If the patient has a hearing loss, a stimulus at 20 dB SL for that patient will not be at the same SPL as a 20 dB SL stimulus presented to a person with normal hearing sensitivity. The SL scale cannot be related to any physical reference until you are informed of the patient's threshold.

The nHL scale refers to stimulus threshold levels that are expected for normal listeners. It is similar, in concept, to the dB hearing level scale used to plot hearing test results. Someone who presents a stimulus at 50 dB nHL is, therefore, presenting it at a level 50 dB above the SPL at which normal listeners first perceive the stimulus.

The only absolute scale among these three commonly employed measures is the SPL scale. The other two require some perceptual measure as a reference point.

SUMMARY

This review of technical aspects of evoked potential recordings has focused on the overall role of the differential preamplifiers and digital averaging systems. The averagers and preamplifiers are required to extract the desired response from background electrical activity. The output of the preamplifier system is influenced strongly by the choice of electrode placement. The nature of the evoked potentials also is influenced by filtering and other procedures used to reduce artifacts and other unwanted noise. Unfortunately, no standard methods have been adopted by individuals reporting on response characteristics, and apparently conflicting results often are due simply to methodology.

Stimuli used for ABR and other evoked potential studies include clicks, tone pips, and tone bursts. Each type of stimulus has its advantages and shortcomings. The click provides the desired abruptness, but offers no well-defined control over stimulus frequency. Tonal stimuli provide better control of frequency, but may sacrifice temporal specificity. Individuals who wish to use the short-latency evoked potentials must recognize the unavoidable interaction between temporal and spectral characteristics of stimuli, and choose stimuli accordingly.

The amplitudes of stimuli used for evoked potential studies have been expressed relative to three different reference points. The scale that uses an absolute reference point is the SPL scale. The SL scale uses the listener's own threshold as the reference point, and the hearing status of that person must be known if comparisons are to be made among listeners. The nHL scale refers to expected thresholds in a specific laboratory or clinic. The absolute SPL corresponding to 0 dB nHL may vary among clinics, but it will be approximately 35 dB SPL when standard earphones are used to conduct the testing.

This chapter concludes our review of basic principles and methods. The remaining chapters will deal with data obtained from normal listeners and clinical patients, and will begin with a consideration of the basic data that pertain to electrocochleography, or the analysis of cochlear and auditory nerve responses.

5

NORMAL COCHLEAR AND AUDITORY NERVE RESPONSES FROM HUMANS

Information regarding human cochlear and auditory nerve responses has been accumulating since the pioneering efforts of Portmann, Yoshie, and their colleagues in the late 1960s. The Electrocochleography supplement of *Acta Oto-laryngologica* (Eggermont et al., 1974) and the collection of research papers under the same title edited by Ruben, Elberling, and Salomon (1976) are important sources of basic information and should be consulted by students who wish to progress beyond the introductory level. Recalling the discussion of earlier chapters, the stimulus-related cochlear potentials (CM and SP) become evident as soon as the eliciting stimulus arrives at the ear. Because they have little or no latency, only the threshold and amplitude characteristics of the CM and SP are available for possible scrutiny. Analysis of the whole nerve AP includes response latency and waveform characteristics in addition to threshold and amplitude information as possible foundations for clinical interpretation.

A major factor influencing the collection of responses from the cochlea and auditory nerve has been the location of the active recording electrode. Popular recording sites for human subjects have included several locations between the cochlear promontory (bone covering the basal turn) and the earlobe. Portmann, LeBert, and Aran (1967) and Yoshie, Ohashi, and Suzuki (1967) independently developed the *transtympanic membrane* technique for obtaining responses from the cochlear promontory. This technique requires that a fine-gauge needle be passed through the tympanic membrane. The needle is held in place by an elastic band that is anchored to a circumaural cushioned ring. Although there have been reports of successful use of the transtympanic membrane electrode with patients who received only a mild sedative most persons using the technique place the electrode only after a local anesthetic has been used in the ear canal. Very young individuals or persons who will not be able to cooperate must be provided with a general anesthesia. Use of the general anesthesia increases the patient risk slightly and markedly increases the cost of the evaluation. Because of these factors and the potential for a transtympanic membrane electrode to cause damage to the middle ear apparatus, many individuals have sought to use less invasive recording procedures.

Yoshie and Yamaura (1969), Coats and Dickey (1970), and Salomon and Elberling (1971) present data obtained with electrodes that were placed beneath the skin of the anesthetized ear canal. This technique avoids risk to the integrity of the tympanic membrane and middle ear, but may require the patient be sedated or be given a general or local anesthetic. Cullen et al. (1972) reported the use of a ball-tipped wire electrode that was placed in contact with the skin of the external meatus near the tympanic membrane. Coats (1974, 1978) and Klein and Mills (1981) have used surface electrodes, placed in the external meatus and held there by plastic leaf or polyethylene tube "springs."

The usual ear-canal surface electrode makes only fair contact with the skin, and its impedance often is in excess of 20,000 ohms. The "reference" electrode attached to the mastoid or earlobe has a normal impedance. This imbalance frequently causes the raw recording to be extremely noisy. The automatic "artifact-reject" feature available on commercial averagers usually will have to be defeated to allow the computer to sample the noisy recording. Adequate ear-canal recordings can be obtained reliably if the following steps are taken: (1) clean the canal of cerumen; (2) dehydrate the skin of the canal with alcohol irrigation; (3) use a generous amount of low-viscosity electrode cream (not paste) on the electrode; and (4) place the electrode within 2 to 3 mm of the tympanic annulus.

The least invasive of the electrodes reported to record cochlear and auditory nerve responses successfully are simple disks that are attached to the earlobe (Sohmer and Feinmesser, 1967; Moore, 1971). The surface electrodes do not require anesthesia and the necessary patient co-operation usually can be obtained voluntarily or with minimal sedation.

The trade-off between patient risk and electrode site is obvious. Unfortunately, the distant recording sites are accompanied by a loss of sensitivity and a complex interaction between recording site and response characteristics. Moving the recording site from the promontory to the earlobe reduces the amplitude of the responses by a factor of about 100. This means that the responses that are as large as 10 μv when recorded from the promontory will be detected as 0.1 μv potentials at the most distal sites. The decrease in magnitude of the response is accompanied by an increase in background noise and an elevation of the response threshold. In our experience, well-placed ear-canal electrodes elicit responses in the range of 0.5 to 2 μv, or about ¹⁄₁₀ the amplitude of the promontory-based recordings. The ear-canal placement corresponds with a threshold sensitivity loss of about 20 dB when compared with the promontory recordings.

There is also an interaction among recording site, stimulus frequency composition, and the relative amplitudes of the various responses (Weiss and Peake, 1972; Durrant and Ronis, 1975; Peck, 1979). For example, Eggermont (1976a) provides examples of marked changes in CM amplitude as the electrode is moved about the promontory surface. Weiss and Peake (1972) noted complex interactions between stimulus frequency and CM amplitude when recording from the cat middle ear. Durrant and Ronis (1975) and Peck (1979) observed changes in the relative amplitudes of the N_1 and N_2 peaks of the AP responses when the recording sites and stimulus characteristics were changed. All of these sources of variability make it difficult to specify absolute norms applicable to measures of the amplitude of the cochlear SP and CM and of the whole nerve AP response. Cochlear responses may dominate the recording when high-intensity stimulation is used and recordings are obtained from the round window or portions of the promontory. Also, the cochlear responses are severely attenuated when recordings are obtained from the more distal sites, and the AP response tends to dominate those records.

Regardless of the recording site, one can identify and separate the cochlear from neural responses by a combination of several techniques that derive from the response characteristics described earlier. It should be recalled that:

The SP is a *dc potential*, usually negative, that accompanies the stimulus, has essentially no latency, and is not masked by the presence of noise or other competing signals.

The CM is an *ac potential* with minimal latency, does not habituate to low and moderate stimulus intensities, and can be obscured, but not masked, by competing signals.

The whole nerve AP has a complex waveform that lags behind the onset of the stimulus and has a waveform, amplitude, and latency that interact with the stimulus characteristics in a complex way. The AP response reveals habituation to rapid stimulus presentation and it can be eliminated by presenting a masking noise along with the stimulus.

If one wishes to reduce the contribution of the AP response in a given recording situation, one could use a stimulus with a slow rise time, repeat the stimulus very rapidly (100 to 200 times per second), or mix the stimulus with a masking noise. The cochlear microphonic may be eliminated by using stimuli of alternating polarity (see Figure 2.3) and the averaging techniques described earlier, or by using a stimulus having a "random" phase, such as a series of noise bursts. It is possible to isolate the summating potential by using rapid stimulus presentations (reducing the AP) or alternating polarity (reducing the CM). An example of the elimination of the CM response to a click stimulus is illustrated in Figure 5.1. The upper tracings show combined CM/AP/SP responses to condensation and rarefaction clicks. The lowest tracing is the SP/AP combination that results from adding the two upper tracings together.

Additional isolation techniques are extensions of these procedures. For example, if one wishes to eliminate the SP and the CM from a recording, one may do so by first collecting responses to alternating stimuli at low repetition rates. This results in a combined SP and AP response. Subsequently, the "pure" SP obtained by using rapid alternating stimuli could be subtracted from the SP/AP combination to produce a clear AP response. The CM can be isolated through a technique that employs manipulation of both the stimulus and response recording polarities, as illustrated in Figure 5.2. The combined CM/SP/AP response is obtained for a fixed-phase stimulus. The upper tracing illustrates this result. The phase of the stimulus then is reversed and the noninverting and inverting inputs to the recording preamplifier are exchanged (or the computer is instructed to invert the response polarity). The result of this dual inversion is illustrated in the bottom tracing. Since the CM was first inverted by the selection of phase of the stimulus and then inverted again by the preamplifier (or computer) it has the same phase as in the top tracing. The AP and SP polarities were affected only by the preamplifier and so they are now the complement of the top tracing. If the result of the top tracing is added to the result of the middle tracing in the computer memory, the combination produces the bottom tracing, consisting of a

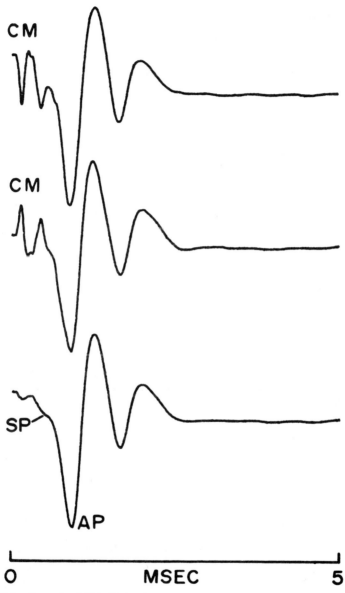

Figure 5.1. Example of CM elimination with preservation of the SP and AP. The upper tracing is a response to condensation clicks. The middle tracing resulted from rarefaction clicks. Note the reversal of the CM. The bottom tracing is the mean of the upper and middle tracings.

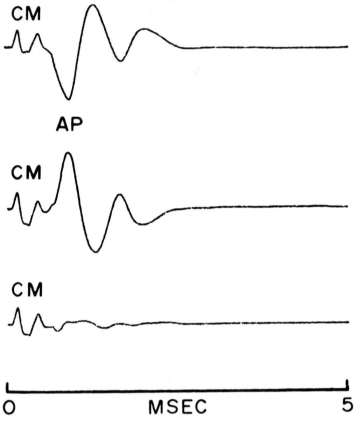

Figure 5.2.   Isolation of the CM response. Both the stimulus and the recording polarities were reversed for the middle tracing. The bottom tracing is the mean of the top and middle responses.

microphonic response. The bottom tracing reveals the mean of the CM voltages.

MEASURES USED TO QUANTIFY THE RESPONSE

Fundamental measurements of the amplitude of the cochlear response and the amplitude/latency of the AP are illustrated in Figure 5.3. The SP measurement is taken as the difference (μv) between the prestimulus baseline and the inflection point on the leading edge of the AP response. Gibson, Moffat, and Ramsden (1977) and Moffat (1979) proposed that the SP magnitude be expressed by the *duration* of the combined SP/AP response, rather than a simple amplitude measurement. Measurements

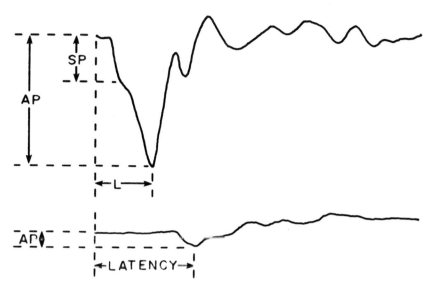

Figure 5.3.   Elementary measures of the SP and AP responses. The upper tracing shows a response to a midintensity stimulus and the lower tracing corresponds to a near-threshold stimulus.

of the amplitude of the CM typically are made in the form of simple peak-to-peak voltages. A more sophisticated approach to examination of the CM in humans was described recently by Hoke (1976). This involved the measurement of the phase of the CM associated with changes in the SPL of the stimulus.

The AP responses are characterized by their latency and amplitude measures, as illustrated in Figure 5.3. The AP amplitude is the voltage difference between the prestimulus baseline and the most negative (N_1) peak of the response. The latency of the response is referenced to either the onset of the computer sampling period or to the time at which the stimulus arrives at the ear. The absolute difference between these two reference points should be 130 to 200 μsec for click stimuli. Estimation of the AP response latency can be accomplished reliably at moderate and high stimulus levels because the response peak is relatively narrow. Near-threshold response latencies sometimes are difficult to specify, however, because the AP has a relatively broad waveform. Estimating the latency as the time delay to the center of the broadened peak seems to be a reasonable approach to this.

The frequency composition and SPL of the stimulus both influence the characteristics of the responses. When promontory-based recordings are obtained, the CM threshold is at 50 to 70 dB SL in normal listeners, and grows directly with SPL until reaching a saturation point at 90 to

100 dB SL (Beagley and Gibson, 1978). The SP follows a similar course, making its first appearance at midintensities and reaching a saturation point around 90 dB SL in normal listeners (Eggermont, 1976b). The same general trends are noted from records obtained with electrodes in the ear canal, but the absolute amplitudes are reduced and one finds a corresponding elevation of response threshold.

A major problem associated with applying measurements of the cochlear potentials to clinical diagnosis stems from their variability across subjects. For example, Hoke (1976) reported that the growth of the CM with changes in stimulus SPL for normal subjects correlates well only for mid- and high-frequency stimuli. Aran and Charlet de Sauvage (1976) report very large standard deviations for CM responses to clicks. Eggermont (1976b) noted that the SP amplitudes exhibited a 10-fold range for midintensity stimulation with tone bursts in normal listeners.

One of the factors that contribute to the variability of the measured amplitudes is the status of the ear under test. A certain amount of variability is expected for ears that appear to be normal on routine audiometrics because of the insensitivity of conventional hearing tests to subtle differences in hearing. However, the large differences found for normal listeners probably reflect such factors as bone structure and precise location of the recording electrode. Isolating sources of variability in the recording would require procedures that are much more time-consuming and invasive than those presently employed and would be impractical to apply routinely. As a result, estimations of the locus or type of cochlear disorder often cannot be made on the basis of cochlear potentials obtained from an individual patient. Large groups of patients fitting a diagnostic category can sometimes be separated by statistical manipulation, but this may not be helpful when one must consider an individual case. One promising attempt at controlling for the nonauditory factors that influence CM and SP response characteristics is to consider the cochlear response amplitudes with reference to the *amplitude* of the AP under standard stimulus conditions in a given patient. In the absence of disorder of the auditory nerve, the whole nerve AP response amplitude can serve as a predictor of *expected* values of the cochlear potentials for high-intensity stimulation (Coats, 1981).

Growth of the AP response in a normal subject with changes in the SPL of a click stimulus is illustrated in Figure 5.4. The amplitude of the response is plotted on two coordinate systems. Figure 5.4A uses the *absolute amplitude* of the AP response and represents that amplitude on a logarithmic scale. Figure 5.4B expresses the amplitude using a *relative* scale. The use of the absolute scale is convenient for purposes of comparing a single subject's responses to various stimuli, such as tone bursts at different frequencies. The plot of relative amplitudes permits com-

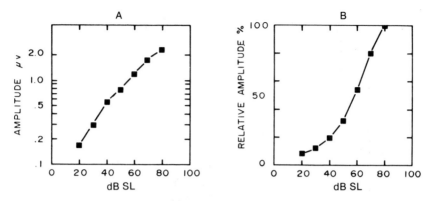

Figure 5.4. Whole nerve AP amplitude for a normal listener expressed in absolute *(A)* and relative *(B)* values. The vertical scale on coordinate system *A* is logarithmic.

parisons across subject groups, recording sites, etc. Note that the normal growth pattern for the AP response has two distinct portions. The near-threshold response grows relatively slowly with increments in stimulus SPL. The response passes through a transition point at about 50 to 60 dB above threshold in normal listeners, and then climbs rapidly toward its maximal amplitude. (The logarithmic scale in Figure 5.4*A* tends to obscure this trend because the vertical scale distance from 0.1 to 1.0 μv is the same as the distance from 1.0 to 10.0 μv.) While the data in Figure 5.4 were obtained using click stimuli, similar patterns are observed for abrupt tonal stimuli. Lower-frequency stimuli tend to elicit responses that are consistently smaller than those obtained for higher frequencies or clicks (Eggermont, 1976a; Zerlin and Naunton, 1976).

The AP response latency is quite stable across recording sites. A normal response latency for near-threshold click stimuli is approximately 4.5 msec. The latency decreases with increases in stimulus SPL and reaches 1.5 to 2.0 msec for stimuli at 80 to 90 dB above threshold. The stability of the latency of the AP response has made it a very attractive measure upon which to determine aberrations in clinical populations. An example of normal response latency for click stimulation is provided in Figure 5.5. Stimulus frequency composition has a major effect on latency. Lowering the frequency corresponds with an increase in response latency, as one would anticipate based on the development of the travelling wave in the cochlea. Zerlin and Naunton (1976) report that the latency increases approximately 3 to 3.5 msec as one changes stimulus frequency from 8,000 Hz to 250 Hz and maintains a constant stimulus SL (65 dB) in normal listeners.

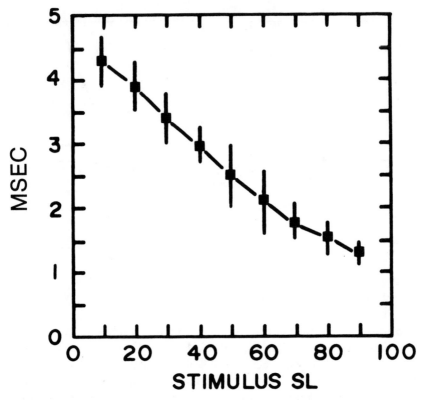

Figure 5.5.   AP response latency for click stimuli. The symbols represent mean data and the vertical bars correspond to the standard deviation for eight normal subjects.

SUMMARY

Taken together, the cochlear and auditory nerve responses that are accessible to the clinical investigator provide very sensitive indices of the status of the auditory periphery. Measures of the absolute amplitude of the SP and CM are highly variable. Records of the AP response obtained from the cochlear promontory have stable amplitudes across subjects, but are quite variable when obtained from the external meatus. Fortunately the stability of the latency of the AP response, regardless of recording site, makes it very attractive as a clinical measurement tool.

Several stimulus and other experimental factors that are known to influence the CM, SP, and AP responses have not been reviewed in this chapter, although the major factors relevant to clinical practice have been described. The interested reader should review the work of Dallos (1973) and other literature cited earlier in this chapter for additional information. Readers interested primarily in the ABR should be certain to inform themselves about the normal and abnormal latency characteristics of the AP, as they can be expected to affect the ABR significantly. Clinical findings based on cochlear and AP responses will be reviewed in Chapter 6.

6

CLINICAL
APPLICATIONS
OF COCHLEAR
AND AUDITORY
NERVE RESPONSES

The principal applications of measures of cochlear and auditory nerve responses lie in the areas of audiometric threshold estimation and site-of-lesion testing. In general, an analysis of the AP response characteristics forms the basis for audiometric impressions, and consideration of the AP as well as the cochlear potentials contributes to the impression of site of lesion.

AUDIOMETRIC THRESHOLD ESTIMATION

Estimations of the threshold of hearing based upon the AP response depend on the examiner's ability to obtain recordings of sufficient sensitivity. The sensitivity of the recording is determined by such factors as electrode location and the temporal characteristics of the stimulus. It should be recalled that the temporal characteristics of the stimulus also determine the frequency specificity of that stimulus (see Figure 3.5.). Unfortunately, the optimal stimulus from the standpoint of the sensitivity of the recording, the click, is the poorest from the perspective of one who wishes to obtain information about the audiogram. Tones of long duration with gradual rise times that provide valid audiometric information generally are poor choices for eliciting the AP. The following three approaches to audiometric estimates are based on the AP response:

Click stimuli are used to determine response threshold in SPL or nHL and characteristics of the suprathreshold responses are examined.
Abrupt tonal stimuli, selected to span the conventional audiometric range, are used to obtain response thresholds.
Using a combination of click stimuli and band-limited noise, "derived" responses are produced in an attempt to parcel the broad cochlear stimulation due to clicks into individual frequency-specific components.

When clicks are employed as stimuli, the agreement between the AP threshold and audiometric thresholds is fair to good in the mid- and high-frequency region. Aran, Charlet de Sauvage, and Pelerin (1971) compared the average hearing loss (250 through 8,000 Hz) to the AP threshold in more than 100 cases and found that the AP tended to *overestimate* slight and mild hearing loss. The prediction from AP to audiometric average was most accurate when the hearing loss exceeded 70 to 80 dB HL. Yoshie (1973) and Eggermont (1976a) examined the correlation between click-elicited AP response threshold and the hearing loss at several individual audiometric frequencies. Their findings suggested that the best correlation could be expected in the region of 2,000 Hz. This is quite understandable on the basis of the information presented in Chapter 3. The estimation of hearing loss based on click stimuli will be insensitive to low-frequency thresholds (Brackmann and Selters, 1976; Glattke, 1978) and its sensitivity to high-frequency hearing will be determined by the shape of the audiogram in the high-frequency region. For example, if the hearing loss were confined to the extreme high-frequency region, one might expect the *latency* of the AP response to reflect the loss of the basal portion of the cochlea. Coats (1978) has reported that the latency of the AP responses increased with the amount of hearing loss in the 4,000 to 8,000 Hz region. This observation suggests that the examination of suprathreshold response latency characteristics, as well as threshold data, may improve the audiometric estimates based on click stimulation.

Obviously, a more direct approach to the use of AP recordings for audiometric purposes involves stimuli that are more frequency-specific than the broad-spectrum clicks. Yoshie (1973) examined the relationship between audiometric thresholds and thresholds for AP responses elicited by tone pips and found correlations approaching 0.9 for the 2 to 8 kHz region. Eggermont, Spoor, and Odenthal (1976) have presented a group of audiograms that show their patients' subjective pure tone thresholds and tone burst AP response thresholds. There is impressive agreement among the thresholds produced by the two techniques, especially in the 2 to 8 kHz region. A summary of their data, which compares audiometric and AP thresholds for the 500 to 8,000 Hz range, suggests mean differences between the two techniques to be always within one audiometric step (5 dB), with standard deviations ranging from 9 to 15 dB. Naunton and Zerlin (1978) reported AP threshold/behavioral comparisons for normal listeners and subjects with hearing loss. Their technique resulted in an overestimation of hearing loss in the 500 to 1,000 Hz range, good agreement at 2,000 Hz, and an underestimation of hearing loss at 8,000 Hz. Coats, Martin, and Kidder (1979) studied the AP responses obtained for tone pips ranging from 250 through 8,000 Hz in five normal subjects. Their recordings were obtained from electrodes placed in the external meatus, whereas the other studies cited previously used transtympanic membrane electrodes. The data from Coats and his coworkers suggest discrepancies between subjective and AP thresholds that range to 50 dB or more as the stimulus frequency is lowered from 8,000 to 250 Hz. Excellent agreement was noted at 8,000 Hz, and the error increased about 10 dB for each octave step downward to 250 Hz.

One concern associated with the use of tone burst or tone pip stimulation for the purpose of estimating audiometric configuration arises from the fact that high-intensity stimulation of the ear results in the production of responses within the basal portion of the cochlea, regardless of the frequency composition of the stimulus (see Chapter 3). In order to create a stimulus situation that would prevent the basal region of the cochlea from contributing to the AP response, several investigators have employed high-frequency *masking noise*. The first study of this type was reported by Teas, Eldredge, and Davis (1962), and it has given rise to the concept of derived frequency-specific responses. The derived response technique requires several steps:

1. The AP response to a click is obtained without any intentional masking noise. This response reflects widespread activation of the cochlea and auditory nerve.
2. Broadband noise is introduced with the click and the level of the noise is adjusted to a value at which it is sufficient just to mask the AP response.
3. The noise is maintained at the SPL determined in step 2, but it is then led through a high-pass filter with a variable cutoff frequency.

The high-pass noise prevents a *restricted* region of the cochlea from participating in the response, and thereby introduces a controlled "hearing loss."

4. The click is reintroduced and an AP response is obtained for the click-plus-narrowband noise combination. An example of responses obtained in this fashion is illustrated in Figure 6.1.

5. The cutoff frequency of the noise then is lowered, so that the effect of the noise spreads to the more apical region of the cochlea. Another AP response is obtained. This step is repeated with successive lowering of the noise cutoff frequency.

6. The individual responses then are subtracted from each other. Examples of the subtraction process are illustrated in the right column of Figure 6.1.

Examination of the responses in the left column of Figure 6.1 reveals that they behave in a manner predicted by the description of cochlear

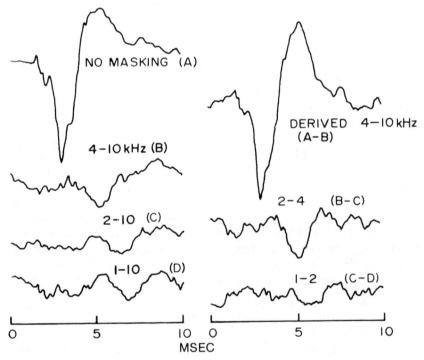

Figure 6.1.   Examples of derived whole nerve action potentials. The left column shows APs obtained under quiet conditions *(A)* and in the presence of bands of noise extending from 10 to 4 kHz *(B)*; 10 to 2 kHz *(C)*; and 10 to 1 kHz *(D)*. The tracings on the right are the computed differences between the individual responses on the left, and reveal the response components that were removed by the extension of the masking noise.

function provided in Chapter 2. Responses obtained with progressive extension of the noise toward the lower-frequency region appear with a progressive increase in latency and a reduction of amplitude. When the subtraction technique of step 6 is employed, one can examine the differences among the masked responses in a more systematic way. The column on the right illustrates the differences between the unmasked and the 4-kHz high-pass masked response, the difference between the 4-kHz and the 2-kHz masked responses, and the difference between the 2-kHz and the 1-kHz masked responses. These *difference tracings* are the derived responses. They reveal components of the response waveform that were removed by each extension of the noise. Early applications of this technique in human subjects (Glattke, 1972; Elberling, 1974; Simmons and Glattke, 1975; Eggermont, Spoor, and Odenthal, 1976; Parker and Thornton, 1978a, 1978b, 1978c) explored its use with both moderate- and high-intensity stimuli.

The clinical application of this technique involves the determination of derived response thresholds for a variety of frequency ranges. The extension of the noise into a *region of hearing loss* will have little effect on the response, and little or no derived response will be detected. For example, if an ear had a steep loss confined to 4,000 Hz and above, adding noise to the 4 to 10 kHz region would not be expected to modify the unmasked response from that ear, and no derived high-frequency response would be found. The derived response is found when the masker extends into a frequency region that had been contributing to the unmasked response. More recently, Don, Eggermont, and Brackmann (1979) have extended this approach to measure threshold levels across the audiometric range for the ABR. The procedure, while time-consuming, predicts audiometric configuration with better accuracy than can be accomplished through the use of abrupt tone bursts or tone pips alone.

In sum, audiometric information obtained through the use of cochleographic techniques is based upon the interpretation of the threshold and latency characteristics of the whole nerve response. Excellent correspondence between audiometric thresholds and whole nerve responses has been reported when promontory-based recordings were used to obtain the AP response, but the ear-canal recordings do not appear to be satisfactory for the purpose of estimating audiometric thresholds below 4,000 Hz. A fundamental problem associated with the use of any tonal stimuli to elicit the AP response is the interaction between intensity and place of stimulation in the cochlea. The interpretation of audiometric thresholds based on click stimuli must be limited to the high-frequency portion of the audiogram regardless of the intensity at which threshold is reached.

SITE-OF-LESION INTERPRETATION

The AP response threshold, growth pattern, latency characteristics, and general waveform have all been implicated as valuable contributors to the localization of the site of the lesion. The discussion that follows is organized around characteristics of the responses that might contribute to a differential diagnosis.

Response Threshold   The response threshold of the AP should, of course, be a fair indicator of the hearing loss within the frequency region of the stimulus used to elicit the response. When the AP response threshold is *much better* than one would anticipate on the basis of the audiogram, the examiner must consider two quite different alternatives: functional hearing loss versus retrocochlear disorders. The utility of the AP response threshold in the identification of exaggerated hearing loss should be self-evident. However, the AP response may also be normal in cases of acoustic neuroma or other space-occupying lesions that involve the auditory nerve (Brackmann and Selters, 1976; Gibson and Beagley, 1976; Coats, 1978; Selters and Brackmann, 1979; Eggermont, Don, and Brackmann, 1980; Portmann et al., 1980). Portmann et al. (1980) suggest that whole nerve AP thresholds that are better than would be expected on the basis of the audiogram are " . . .the strongest indicator of a retrocochlear disorder . . ." (p. 365). In their group of 14 tumor patients, four presented AP thresholds better than suggested by audiometric information. Eggermont, Don, and Brackmann (1980) report AP threshold abnormalities in only 8% of their tumor cases. The Brackmann and Selters (1976) report included one case of complete deafness (through 8,000 Hz) associated with AP responses that were normal in every respect. While the alternatives faced by the diagnostician confronted with a hearing loss by audiometric testing and normal AP responses are quite distinct, they have a common basis. Cochlear and peripheral nerve integrity are, of course, intact in the case of functional hearing loss. Apparently, the space-occupying lesions causing hearing loss will also leave the periphery intact in some significant number of tumor patients, as well.

Response Growth Patterns   The patterns of response growth are quite sensitive to the presence of cochlear pathology. The most common finding in the case of cochlear disorder is the *recruiting* growth pattern. Examples of a recruiting pattern are illustrated in Figure 6.2 (cf. Eggermont, 1976a; Yoshie, 1976; Glattke, 1978; and others). The normal AP growth, when plotted on a relative amplitude scale, passes through gradual and steep slope regions. The recruiting pattern is characterized by

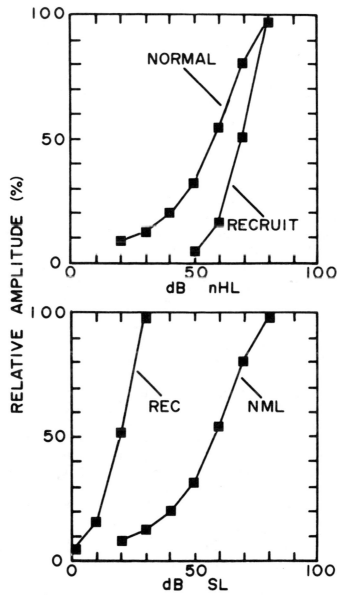

Figure 6.2.   Example of normal and recruiting AP response growth patterns. The response amplitudes in the upper graph are plotted against an nHL scale. The lower graph shows the same data plotted against an SL scale to emphasize the steep growth pattern of the recruiting response.

an elevated threshold and a rapid ascent to maximum amplitude once the stimulus exceeds threshold. The recruiting pattern is, therefore, very similar to the high-intensity portion of the normal response curve. The distinct nature of the recruiting pattern is best illustrated when it is plotted in against the listener's own threshold for the stimulus, as in the lower graph of Figure 6.2. The other major finding regarding AP amplitude is the response that fails to grow into the normal amplitude range, even though the stimulus may reach 30 to 50 dB above the patient's hearing loss. (This finding would be obscured by the use of the relative amplitude plots of Figure 6.2, since the response amplitude must always reach 100%.) One cause of this effect is conductive hearing loss. If the conductive loss includes the high-frequency region and extends to 50 or 60 dB on a conventional audiogram, the stimulus would not reach the cochlea with sufficient intensity to develop the normal high-intensity response growth. There are few reports of substantial pure conductive loss in the literature concerning cochleography (Eggermont, 1976a). A practical reason for this is that the physical findings upon otoscopic evaluation in the case of moderate to severe conductive loss would be so obvious that electrophysiologic studies would not be required to arrive at a diagnosis.

The second major cause of AP responses with reduced amplitude is severe hearing loss, regardless of site of lesion. (This has an obvious cause and effect, but the fact that the relationship between severe hearing loss and poor definition of the AP response is obvious should not preclude the examination of AP responses in cases of severe unilateral loss. As noted previously, normal AP responses in those cases suggest a retrocochlear lesion.) The final possibility that must be evaluated by a diagnostician confronted with no or minimal AP response amplitudes to high-intensity stimulation is, of course, retrocochlear disorder. Eggermont, Don, and Brackmann (1980) report that 8% of 32 patients with tumors tested by cochleography exhibited abnormal AP growth patterns, although it is unclear whether those same patients also had the greatest hearing losses.

Response Latencies and Hearing Loss   Examples of responses obtained for click stimuli in the case of one normal listener and two individuals with high-frequency loss are illustrated in Figure 6.3. When click stimuli are used and the hearing loss involves the high-frequency region, the near-threshold response latencies tend to be prolonged. The latencies decrease rapidly toward normal values as the stimulus is increased in SPL. When plotted as in Figure 6.4, the latencies are ordered according to the amount of threshold shift. Coats (1978) has reported that the relationship between amount of high-frequency hearing loss and

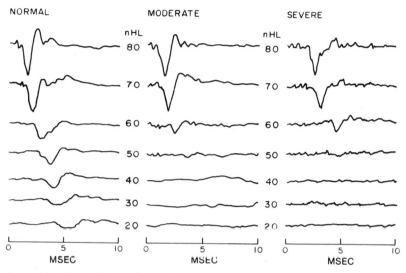

Figure 6.3   Examples of click-elicited AP responses in cases of moderate and severe high-frequency hearing loss.

AP response latency is so strong that it may preclude identification of site of lesion. This follows from the fact that serious cochlear disorder often accompanies the presence of a retrocochlear problem, and the influence of the cochlear disorder is so strong that the retrocochlear effects are obscured by the hearing loss. In an exception to this general finding, Eggermont (1976a) reports that the AP response latencies for ears having retrocochlear disorders may reveal irregularities in their latency/intensity functions if midfrequency (2,000 Hz) tone bursts are used to elicit the responses. Eggermont (1976a) suggests that it is a waveform abnormality that influences the response latency measurement in the case of the retrocochlear patients. If one takes the center of the broadened waveform as the point at which latency is measured, then the resulting measurement will be prolonged. In an attempt to describe subtle differences caused by alterations of the waveform of the response, Eggermont (1976a) and his coworkers (Odenthal and Eggermont, 1976) have examined response amplitude as a function of response latency for normal subjects and groups of patients with hearing loss. The results from the patients diagnosed as having Ménière's disease were indistinguishable from the normal population. Approximately 60% of the data points for patients with cochlear (non-Ménière) hearing loss were outside of the normal range because the responses tended to be of *brief latency* but of normal amplitude. About 40% of their patients with retrocochlear tumors clustered in the opposite direction, with *prolonged latencies*. Pro-

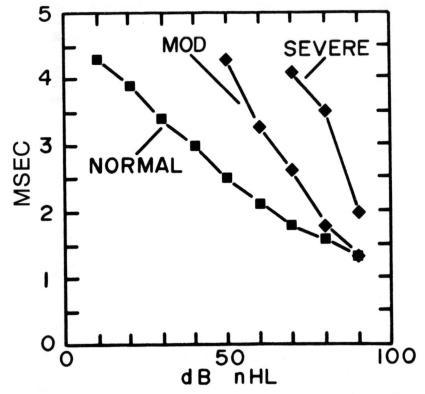

Figure 6.4.   Examples of AP response latency characteristics with various degrees of hearing loss.

longations also have been noted for patients with multiple sclerosis (Parving, Elberling, and Smith, 1981). Sometimes, cerebral vascular accidents may produce changes in the AP response (Nishida, Kumagami, and Baba, 1981).

Aberrations of the Response Waveform   Response waveform aberrations are suggested as indices of site of lesion by a number of investigators (Yoshie and Ohashi, 1969; Aran, Charlet de Sauvage, and Pelerin, 1971; Portmann and Aran, 1972; Yoshie, 1973, 1976). The aberrations appear to be of two types: those that clearly involve a modification of the *neural response*, and those that provide a peculiar configuration due to the presence of an enlarged *summating potential*. AP responses that are not contaminated by the SP include those obtained from patients with retrocochlear lesions by Portmann and Aran (1972), who described "larges" (broad) responses for individuals having a variety of etiologies, including metabolic disorders and space-occupying lesions. Brackmann and Selters (1976) provide examples of AP responses for 16 tumor patients. Their examples are reproduced in Figure 6.5, and, as can be determined from the illustration, the responses range from broad and indistinct waveforms to normal. About 70% of the patients with Ménière's disease presented by Brackmann and Selters had abnormal response waveforms. The most common AP response abnormality in those cases was a multiple-peaked response, a result similar to that reported by Odenthal and Eggermont (1976).

Summating Potential   The SP contributes to abnormal response waveforms in a significant number of cases of Ménière's disease (Eggermont, 1976b; Odenthal and Eggermont, 1976; Gibson et al., 1977; Eggermont, 1979; Moffat, 1979; Coats, 1981). There have been a few reports of an SP response that has a positive polarity (Aran, 1971; Yoshie,

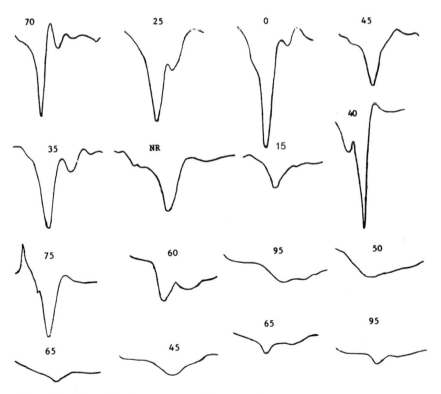

Figure 6.5.   Examples of response waveforms in 16 tumor patients. The number above each response is the patient's hearing threshold at 4 kHz. Reprinted with permission from Brackmann and Selters (1976).

1976), but most reports have dealt with the effects of a negative SP. Two characteristics of the SP, its duration and amplitude, appear to be most promising as candidates for classification of the SP abnormalities. The "width" measure advocated by Moffat (1979) expresses the duration of the response from the onset of the SP/AP complex until the waveform returns to the voltage measured as the prestimulus baseline. Because the SP normally mimics the envelope of the stimulus, its duration should equal the stimulus duration. Moffat noted durations of the SP that varied over a range of about 2 to 9 msec in repeated studies of a patient with Ménière's disease. Eggermont (1976b) examined the ratio of the SP amplitude to the AP response for patients grouped as normals, Ménière, and cochlear (non-Ménière). Using tone bursts of 2, 4, and 8 kHz, he found considerable overlap of the ratio of SP and AP measures obtained for his various groups of subjects. For high stimulus levels, the SP/AP amplitude ratio was about 0.4 for the patients with Ménière's disease and slightly less for the other groups. A clearer separation of Ménière and non-Ménière patients was achieved by Coats (1981) using click stimuli presented at a fixed high intensity. A summary of Coats's data is provided in Figure 6.6. The amplitude of the SP was related to the AP amplitude in a complex, curvilinear fashion. The continuous lines in each panel represent functions that are ± 2 standard deviations away from and parallel to a parabolic curve that was a "best fit" for his group of normal ears. The individual datum points correspond to results for patients that fit into the retrocochlear, cochlear (non-Ménière), and Ménière groups. The SP/AP amplitude relationships determined for patients with retrocochlear lesions were indistinguishable from the normal group results, as only a single data point fell outside the normal limits. By

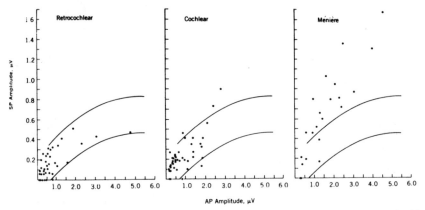

Figure 6.6.   SP/AP amplitude characteristics in three groups of patients. Reprinted with permission from Coats (1981).

contrast, some 68% of the results from patients with Ménière's disease scattered outside the normal boundaries. The data indicate that an increase of SP amplitude is associated with Ménière's disease. Coats also noted that the amplitudes of the CM obtained from the Ménière's patients were consistently larger than those obtained for the other patient groups. This finding is in contrast with the results reviewed by Gibson (1978), who notes that an increased amplitude of the CM, particularly in the presence of a small AP response, may help to pinpoint the presence of a retrocochlear disorder.

The relationships of CM amplitude to site of lesion do not appear to have been documented consistently in the literature. (Some of the probable sources of variability of CM measures were discussed in Chapter 5.) At present, reliance on CM measures without consideration of overall response amplitudes, AP and SP characteristics and other diagnostic information does not seem very promising (cf. Aran and Charlet de Sauvage, 1976; Beagley and Gibson, 1978).

SUMMARY

Table 6.1 summarizes some of the alternative decisions that must be considered by the examiner when any of several common outcomes are encountered. Generally one can expect that the AP thresholds and latencies to be sensitive to peripheral hearing loss. The accuracy with which one can predict audiometric threshold from the AP response threshold is quite good in the high-frequency region, and acceptable in the low- and mid-frequency region when promontory electrodes are used. Threshold estimation based on surface electrodes is adequate for high frequencies only. Response latency characteristics are sensitive to site of lesion and amount of hearing loss. For example, conductive hearing loss that involves the high-frequency region will result in an AP latency-intensity function that is parallel to the normal response curve but exhibits prolonged latencies. Precipitous high-frequency hearing loss also will result in prolonged AP latencies, but in many cases of sensorineural loss the AP latency will approach normal values for high-intensity stimulation. The recruiting aspect of the response amplitude helps to locate the site of lesion in the cochlea. Analysis of the SP has received growing acceptance as a sensitive indicator of cochlear disorders, particularly Ménière's disease.

In overview, the analysis of cochlear and auditory nerve responses provides a very sensitive reflection of the status of the peripheral auditory system, up to the internal auditory meatus. The electrocochleographic methods can be of great diagnostic value. This is particularly true when

Table 6.1. Summary of common electrocochleographic test results and their
related diagnostic alternatives

Test results	Rule out	Possible conclusions
AP is normal with threshold better than audiogram suggests.	Functional hearing loss	Hearing loss is due to retrocochlear disorder.
AP threshold is elevated and the response has a brief latency.	Poor electrode placement	This suggests sensorineural hearing loss but may not be localizing.
AP threshold is elevated and the response latency is prolonged.	Conductive hearing loss	This may occur for severe high-frequency sensorineural hearing loss (regardless of site of lesion).
AP response is aberrant, with multiple peaks or broad waveform.	Stimulus artifact[a]	Broadened waveform may be due to the SP or to retrocochlear sources. Multipeaked responses are associated with Ménière's.
AP amplitude is very small at high stimulus intensities.	Poor electrode placement	Severe high-frequency loss, conductive or retrocochlear disorder must be considered.
AP amplitude is normal in spite of threshold elevation.		This is the recruiting response most often associated with cochlear disorders.
SP/CM are present, but there is no AP response.	Stimulus artifact[a]	This points to retrocochlear disorders.
SP is abnormally large.	Stimulus artifact[a]	This is most often found with Ménière's disease.

[a] Refers to the radiation of the stimulus electrical waveform to the patient electrodes. This will produce a microphoniclike voltage that obscures the desired cochlear or auditory nerve response.

the measures are incorporated into a test protocol that includes the ABR. From an audiometric screening standpoint, the analysis of AP responses may be an important adjunct to ABR threshold studies in patients who are neurologically compromised (Ryerson and Beagley, 1981). In addition, the combination of ABR and electrocochleography appears to offer great sensitivity and precision in the detection of space-occupying lesions that involve the auditory nerve (Eggermont, Don, and Brackmann, 1980).

7

NORMAL AUDITORY BRAINSTEM RESPONSES FROM HUMANS

Jewett and his coworkers provided the earliest complete descriptions of the ABR in both laboratory animals and humans. Jewett, Romano, and Williston (1970) and Jewett and Williston (1971) explored such variables as electrode locations, stimulus repetition rate, and amplifier filter characteristics, and provided the Roman numeral designation for response peaks that has been adopted by many investigators. Sohmer and Zuckerman (1979) have reviewed the peak designations used by a number of investigators, and the interested reader should review their concise summary. The basic data obtained from the ABR consist of measures of latency and amplitude. Typically, amplitude is measured as the difference between a voltage peak and the subsequent negative minimum, or trough, as illustrated in Figure 7.1. Latencies are measured to the peaks that are of interest just as they are for measures of AP latency. Once the latencies of the response peaks have been determined, the intervals between the peaks may be computed simply by subtracting the latency of one peak from the other.

The responses illustrated in Figure 7.1 provide clear examples of the peaks that are of interest. Frequently an examiner will find that either

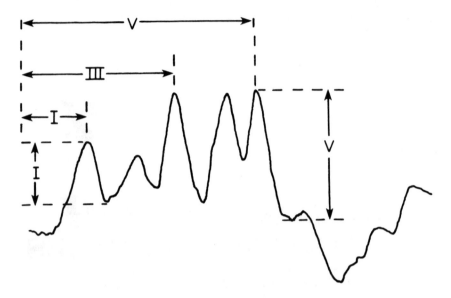

Figure 7.1. Examples of ABR measurement schemes. Latency measures are taken as indicated by the horizontal arrows. Amplitude measures are noted by the vertical arrows.

not all peaks are present or that some peaks appear to have merged. This merging often is encountered for the peaks designated as IV and V. The loss of peaks I, II, and III typically is encountered when the stimulus is at a low SL. Worthington and Peters (1980a) and Rose (in press) have presented data illustrating the probability of detecting peaks I through V for normal listeners at various stimulus SLs. The two studies revealed similar findings in that wave V was detected for 75% or more normal listeners at a threshold of 10 to 20 dB SL, and from virtually all listeners for stimuli exceeding 20 dB SL. According to their data, wave III will first appear in 50 to 60% of normal listeners for stimuli that are presented at 30 dB SL. According to Worthington and Peters, wave I appears in about 75% of the normal population when the stimulus reaches 50 dB SL. Rose's findings suggest that it may appear only in about 50% of the population for stimuli at 70 dB SL. This information is important to those who would use ABR evaluations clinically, because it provides a basis for expectations regarding the thresholds of the individual response peaks in routine practice. The data suggest that one often will not be able to identify waves preceding wave V, even for stimuli of moderate to high intensity.

NORMAL LATENCY OF THE ABR

Table 7.1 provides a summary of the latency of responses published by four laboratories. The data are arranged in columns that correspond to

Table 7.1.   Latencies (in msec) of peaks I through V of the ABR as reported by several laboratories. The measures are listed in rows according to the sensation level or hearing level of the click stimulus. The studies are numbered as follows: (1) Starr and Achor (1975), 10 clicks per second; (2) Rosenhamer, Lindstrom, and Lundborg (1978), 16.6 clicks per second; (3) Beagley and Sheldrake (1978), 20 clicks per second; (4) Rowe (1978) 30 clicks per second.

Stimulus SL or nHL	Wave I				Wave II				Wave III				Wave IV				Wave V			
	Study no.				Study no.				Study no.				Study no.				Study no.			
	1	2	3	4	1	2	3	4	1	2	3	4	1	2	3	4	1	2	3	4
85 to 90			1.3				2.4				3.6				4.9				5.6	
75 to 80	1.4	1.4	1.9		2.6	2.6	3.1		3.7	3.6	4.1		4.6	4.8	5.1		5.4	5.5	5.9	
65 to 70	1.6	1.5			2.8	2.7			3.8	3.7			4.8	4.9			5.5	5.6		
55 to 60	1.8	1.7	2.3	1.96	3.0	2.9	3.4	2.98	3.9	3.9	4.6	4.01	5.0	5.2	5.7	5.19	5.8	5.9	6.4	6.01
45 to 50	2.2				3.3				4.3				5.4				6.0	6.2		
35 to 40	2.7				3.6				4.7				5.8				6.6	6.5		
25 to 30	2.9				3.8				5.1				6.6				7.1	7.0		
15 to 20									5.9								7.7	7.8		
5 to 10									5.6								8.1			

the repetition rate of clicks used to elicit the responses, from 10 through 30 clicks per second. The data of Starr and Achor (1975) were collected from individuals aged 25 to 30 years, using clicks presented at a rate of 10 per second. The data of Rosenhamer, Lindstrom, and Lundberg (1978) were obtained from subjects aged 12 to 40 years, with clicks presented at a rate of 16.6 per second. The data of Beagley and Sheldrake (1978) are from 20-year-old subjects, and their stimulus rate was 20 clicks per second. The data reported by Rowe (1978) were from subjects aged 17 to 33 years, and were based on 30 clicks per second. In spite of differences in rates and recording techniques, the data in the table are remarkably similar and they compare favorably with other data reported by Terkildsen, Osterhammel, and Huis in't Veld (1973), Hecox and Galambos (1974), Pratt and Sohmer (1976), and Coats (1978). The within-laboratory standard deviations of all measures typically range from about 0.16 msec for high-intensity stimulation to larger values for near-threshold responses, which compares favorably with the ranges reported in Table 7.1.

As the data in Table 7.1 reveal, the latency for the major response peaks varies systematically with stimulus SPL. For wave V, this change amounts to 400 to 600 μsec per 10-dB step between 10 and 50 dB SL. The rate of change slows to 100 to 300 μsec per 10-dB step above 60 dB SL. For the click stimuli like those used to obtain the data compiled in the table, the rate of change for the other peak latencies nearly parallels the rate of change for wave V, although differences occur for low-intensity stimulation. The I–III and I–V intervals decrease near threshold. The average intervals among wave I, III, and V latencies summarized in Table 7.1 are listed in Table 7.2 for three ranges of intensity. The intervals are thought to reflect central nervous system processes by most authors and have been called "central transmission time" or "brainstem transmission time" measures (Fabiani et al., 1979). Typically, the interval is about 2 msec for the I–III and III–V intervals, and about 4 msec for the I-V latency difference. As will be discussed in Chapter 8, the intervals between response peaks are very sensitive to the presence of retro-cochlear disorders.

Table 7.2. Average intervals among wave I, III, and V latencies listed in Table 7.1

Stimulus SL or nHL	I–III interval	III–V interval	I–V interval
75 to 80	2.24 msec	1.80 msec	4.04 msec
55 to 60	2.16 msec	1.92 msec	4.08 msec
35 to 40	2.00 msec	1.85 msec	3.85 msec

NORMAL AMPLITUDE OF THE ABR

In contrast to the general agreement regarding response latencies, measures of response amplitude appear to vary greatly. There is a trend for response amplitude to increase directly with stimulus SL, but the absolute amplitudes of individual waves are quite variable. Thornton (1975, 1976) approached this problem by plotting his normative data on coordinates that represented response amplitude on the vertical axis and response component latency on the horizontal axis. The data points are grouped within ellipses corresponding to each response component, reflecting the variability of the response measurements. By providing a range of both amplitude and latency values against which a specific response may be contrasted, Thornton's technique frees the examiner from reliance on a single-point measurement when considering clinical materials. Another approach to the amplitude variability problem is to use a *relative* measurement and consider the amplitude of a specific response component as a ratio percentage or ratio of the amplitude of wave V. Starr and Achor (1975) found that wave V always exceeded the amplitude of wave I in normal subjects. Stockard, Stockard, and Sharbrough (1978) reported that the average ratio of V to I reached 2.5 in the case of normal subjects. The amplitude ratio measures are widely accepted among practitioners. The ratio measures are quite sensitive to factors such as response filtering (see Figure 7.1) and stimulus repetition rate (see Figure 7.2). Someone who wishes to adopt those measures should review the methods used by previous investigators very carefully.

FACTORS AFFECTING THE NORMAL RESPONSE

The morphology (waveform shape), amplitude, and latency of the ABR are influenced by several variables associated with methods of recording and with subject characteristics. Some of the variables reported in the literature are listed in Table 7.3. The following sections of this chapter will review those factors noted in the table.

Rate of Stimulus Presentation Jewett and Williston (1971) described changes in the morphology of the ABR as the stimulus repetition rate was changed from 2.5 to 50 per second, and their findings have been replicated by many other studies. The responses in Figure 7.2 illustrate typical findings, obtained from a normal listener using clicks presented at 60 dB SL and at rates from 10 to 50 per second. All of the first five response components are distinct at 10 per second, but the earliest of them become obscured as the rate is increased. Chiappa, Glad-

Table 7.3.   A partial list of variables influencing the
characteristics of the ABR

Recording methodology	Subject characteristics
Stimulus characteristics	Age
Rate of presentation	Gender
Frequency composition	Body temperature
Onset phase	Drugs
Recording techniques	
Electrode locations	
Filter settings	

stone, and Young (1979) report the "frequency of recognizability" of individual response waves for clicks at a nominal 60 dB SL presented at rates from 10 through 70 per second. They claim that for stimuli presented at 70 per second, wave V was detected in 99% of the records, wave III was detected in 85%, and that wave I was noted in 76%. Pratt and Sohmer (1976) report reductions of amplitude in all response components as the stimulus rate was increased to 80 per second, but they make no mention of encountering any difficulties in recognizing the individual waves. The causes of the changes in response morphology have not been determined exactly. It is doubtful that the selective reduction of the earliest waves represents solely a loss of synchrony or rapid habituation of the auditory nerve. Other factors that probably contribute to the change in response shape include the addition of overlapping electrophysiologic responses having latencies greater than about 10 msec. Changes in the spectra of the click trains associated with changes in repetition rate also influence the response.

The effects of changing stimulus rate on response latency have been reported by a number of investigators. Don, Allen, and Starr (1977) report prolongations of wave V up to 0.9 msec as stimulus rate increases from 10 to 100 per second. Stockard et al. (1979) report a greater prolongation for wave V than for wave I for rates changing between 10 and 80 per second, and, as a result, a change in normal interpeak intervals. Their mean I–V interval increased approximately 0.45 msec when responses to the rapid presentation rates were compared with those at the 10 per second rate. Rosenhamer, Lindstrom, and Lundborg (1978) report no latency shifts for a change of repetition rate from 12.5 to 25 clicks per second.

In sum, it would appear that the threshold and latency of wave V are not seriously compromised by the use of stimulus rates up to about 25 or 30 clicks per second. Wave V persists with a prolonged latency for rates exceeding 30 per second, but there is disagreement in the literature as to the persistence of the other response components. A con-

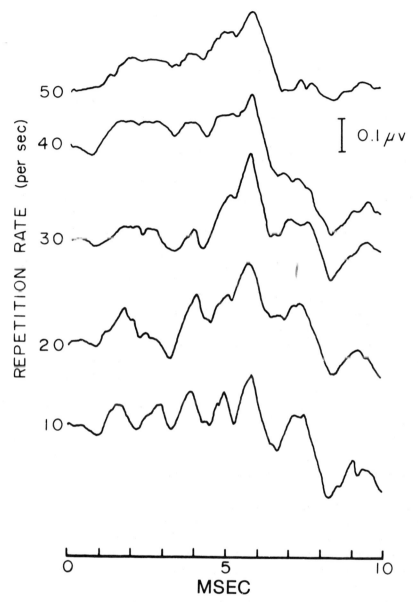

Figure 7.2.   Examples of changes in ABR response characteristics with changes of stimulus repetition rate. The stimulus level was 60 dB SL.

servative approach to testing would suggest the use of low repetition rates when clear measures of waves I, III, and V were desired, whereas high rates (30 per second) would be acceptable for threshold and latency measures that were restricted to wave V.

Stimulus Frequency Composition   The use of tone bursts, tone pips, or derived responses has been reported by a number of investigators. Major studies of derived responses include the work of Parker and Thornton (1978a,b,c), Don and Eggermont (1978), Don, Eggermont, and Brackmann (1979), and Eggermont and Don (1980). The general effect of extending a band of noise from the high-frequency region to lower frequencies is a prolongation of the latencies of the response components. Once the noise band extends into the midfrequency region (about 2,000 Hz), the individual response peaks become less distinct and a single major peak commonly is observed at a prolonged intensity.

Tone pips produce shifts of wave V latency and changes of response morphology similar to those produced by the addition of masking noise. Lowering the frequency of a tone pip is accompanied by a prolongation of the latency of wave V (Klein and Teas, 1978; Terkildsen, Osterhammel, and Huis in't Veld, 1975; Coats, Martin, and Kidder, 1979).

Some studies of the derived response and tone pips report that changes of the response wave characteristics are not exactly parallel when the stimulus properties are changed. According to Coats, Martin, and Kidder (1979), interwave interval measurements based on the whole nerve AP (equivalent to wave I) and wave V reduced to as little as 1.5 msec for 500 Hz tone pips. The latency of the AP response was delayed much more than the latency of wave V as the frequency was lowered to 500 Hz. Measures of amplitudes accompanying changes in frequency (Don and Eggermont, 1978; Eggermont and Don, 1980) of the derived responses also were not parallel across response components. One hypothesis that has emerged from these observations is that the regions of cochlear origin for the processes that generate wave I are different from those that lead to wave V. The origin of wave I may be more basalward than the region that gives rise to wave V. As the frequency of the stimulus (or masking noise) is extended downward, the site(s) move toward the cochlear apex at different rates. A practical implication of this hypothesis is that hearing loss would be expected to have differential effects on wave I and wave V. Hearing loss confined to the high-frequency region may be associated with a greater shift of the latency of wave I than of wave V. Cases of precipitous high-frequency hearing loss would result in a reduction of the interval between I and V. This relationship has been demonstrated by Coats (1978).

Other approaches to identifying frequency selective responses in the early-latency time domains have included the use of tone bursts to elicit the SN-10 response (Davis and Hirsh, 1979; Hawes and Greenberg, 1981; Battmer and Lehnhardt, 1981). Funasaka and Abe (1979) and Glattke (1976) have reported short-latency response characteristics associated with frequency-modulated tonal stimuli.

Phase of Stimulus Onset   Manipulation of the phase of the eliciting stimulus was described previously as a useful technique in the cancellation of the CM or stimulus artifact. One consequence of changing the initial phase of a click stimulus from condensation to rarefaction is a change in the latency of the whole nerve AP response. Stockard et al. (1979) reported statistically significant changes of the intervals between waves I and V and other changes of ABR morphology when the stimulus phase was reversed. Other investigators, however (Terkildsen, Osterhammel, and Huis in't Veld, 1973; Rosenhamer, Lindstrom, and Lund borg, 1978; Coats, 1978), report negligible differences in responses obtained by use of condensation, rarefaction, or alternating click polarities. Coats and Martin (1977) reported complicated interactions between stimulus phase and response morphology when examining patients with varying degrees of hearing loss. Their findings may bear on the discrepancies that have been reported in the literature. Specifically, when the stimulus consists of very high-frequency energy (and the listener's ear is intact) the phase reversal of the click stimulus imposes only a brief functional delay to the moment of neural response generation. This would be predicted as half the period of the highest stimulus frequency that generates the response (e.g., 6 to 8 kHz for high-intensity click stimulation and good quality earphones). If lower frequencies are emphasized, due to earphone characteristics or hearing loss, the effective period of the stimulus will lengthen. This may produce greater differences in the AP response onset latency when the effects of condensation and rarefaction clicks are compared. Variability due to characteristics of earphones and subject status probably contributes to the range of findings in the literature.

Electrode Positions   The electrode positions favored by most investigators of the ABR include one in the skull midline (at the vertex or forward of the vertex) and one ipsilateral to the ear receiving the stimulus (mastoid, earlobe, or neck). The electrodes on the midline and near the ear are coupled to the noninverting and inverting amplifier inputs according to the preference of the investigator. A third, common, electrode is placed on the side of the unstimulated ear or on the forehead. The interaction of electrode site and the differential amplifiers used to detect the responses will produce ABR waveforms that are electrical compromises between the responses detected by the active and reference electrodes. As a consequence, a wide variety of response waveform characteristics have been reported.

Several studies (Jewett and Williston, 1971; Picton et al., 1974; Stockard, Stockard, and Sharbrough, 1978) have examined the effects of moving the reference (inverting) electrode from the stimulated ear to the opposite side. The effects of shifting the inverting electrode from ipsilateral to contralateral mastoid are illustrated in Figure 7.3. Generally, there is a loss of wave I and subtle phase shifts of the other response components. The contralateral reference has been suggested as a site that favors the separation of waves in a blended IV–V complex.

Parametric studies of the effects of electrode positions reported by Terkildsen and Osterhammel (1981) and by Parker (1981) have focused

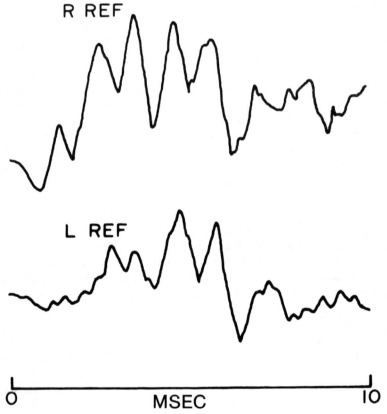

Figure 7.3.   Illustration of the effects of shifting the reference (inverting) electrode from the mastoid ipsilateral (right) to the stimulus ear to the contralateral (left) mastoid.

on optimal recording sites. Terkildsen and Osterhammel explored changes in the ABR with sites that included the neck, earlobes, and vertex in various configurations. They conclude that the earlobe ipsilateral to the stimulus combined with the vertex provides good information for most routine purposes, and suggest that other sites are useful for enhancing certain of the response components, such as wave I. Parker used 16 electrode locations in various combinations and presented the mean and standard deviation values for amplitude and latency measures of waves I, III, and V. Optimal recording sites were different for each of the waves. For example, wave I was best recorded between electrodes placed at the center of the forehead and the mastoid ipsilateral to the stimulus. Wave V was of greatest amplitude with a vertex placement. The optimal placements for detecting all three waves was in the skull midline behind the vertex and the ipsilateral mastoid. A recent study by Prasher and Gibson (1981) included a novel modification of traditional electrode placements. They noted that the ABR seen from an electrode on the mastoid ipsilateral to the stimulus ear had a phase characteristic opposite to that seen on the contralateral mastoid. Prasher and Gibson elected to place the noninverting electrode on one mastoid and the inverting electrode on the contralateral mastoid. Monotic stimulation of each ear separately produced ABRs that were nearly mirror images in terms of response phase, and so binaural stimulation produced responses that effectively cancelled each other. The cancellation will occur only if the waveforms detected from both mastoids are identical, or nearly so, and the procedure should be sensitive to asymmetries of the responses due to hearing loss. Prasher and Gibson report its application as a gross screening technique to detect asymmetry of hearing loss (by simulating conductive hearing loss in normal subjects) and also explored the phenomenon as a correlate to loudness recruitment.

Overall, the literature on electrode placements suggests that the ability to detect individual response components and the apparent phase (apparent latency) of those components will be quite sensitive to electrode location. If one wishes to use published norms regarding response amplitudes and interwave intervals, strict adherence to the methods associated with those norms would seem to be indicated.

Filter Settings   As reviewed in Chapter 4, the filters used with the preamplification system make an important contribution to the reduction of unwanted noise. In the case of ABR recordings, most of the noise is found in the low-frequency region, because it is due to relatively slow electromyographic (EMG) sources. The amplitude of the EMG noise can reach 100 or more times the amplitude of the desired ABR, making elimination of the noise by averaging techniques nearly impossible. If a patient should swallow (and an artifact rejection system is not available) during a sampling epoch, the EMG created by that activity could render the sampling attempt useless.

This problem can be reduced by raising the low-frequency cutoff of the preamplifier to 100 or more Hz. If one raises the low-frequency cutoff above about 50 Hz, the slow-wave portion of the ABR upon which the fast components ride will also be reduced or eliminated. If the high-frequency filter cutoff is lowered below about 3,000 Hz, the fast components will be shifted in phase, and their latencies will change. Examples of the effects of various filter settings on the appearance of the ABR response are illustrated in Figure 7.4, and those examples are representative of the general changes that might be expected. Laukli and Mair (1981) have reported a systematic study of filter effects on the ABR in humans and laboratory animals. They noted that raising the low-frequency cutoff from 2 to 100 Hz resulted in complex changes that included loss of the slow component of the response and a reduction of the apparent latencies of the response peaks. Because the latency reduction was not uniform for all peaks, the interwave intervals were also affected. Lowering the high-frequency cutoff from 5,000 to 1,000 Hz produced increases in the apparent latency of all of the waves of the response.

An important implication of Laukli and Mair's work is that the normative data against which an examiner would compare specific clinical findings must have been collected under the same response filtering conditions as the clinical data. Laukli and Mair do not specify absolute filter settings for routine use, but do recommend a wide filter bandwidth to avoid distortion of the response component amplitudes and latencies. Fria (1980) has reviewed the various filter settings used by a number of investigators and has noted that the preamplifier filter settings of 100 to 3,000 Hz seem to be chosen by most investigators.

EFFECTS OF SUBJECT CHARACTERISTICS

Age   ABRs have been reported for individuals ranging from 26 weeks post-conceptional age (Starr et al., 1977) into the ninth decade of life (Fujikawa and Weber, 1977). Major changes of the morphology, latencies, and thresholds of the responses have been described for those obtained during the first few weeks and months of life. An overview of published evidence suggests that the responses tend to assume characteristics like those obtained from adult subjects when the individuals from whom the responses are obtained reach 18 to 30 months of age.

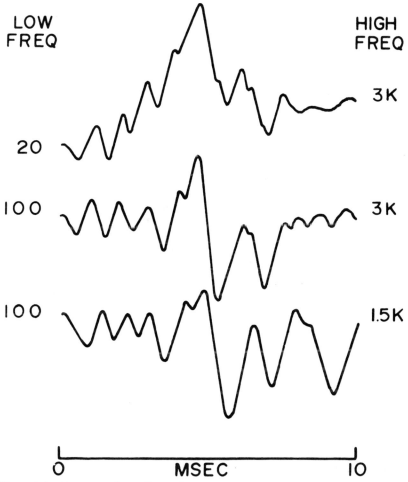

Figure 7.4.   Examples of the effects of altering high- and low-frequency filter settings on the ABR.

Figure 7.5 is an illustration of responses obtained from a normal-term infant. The responses to high-intensity stimulation consist of a multiple-wave ensemble in which the peaks are designated as I, III, and V, as are the peaks in the adult response. Some studies of responses from very young individuals report response waveform characteristics quite similar to those obtained from adult listeners (Salamy, McKean, and Buda, 1975; Starr et al., 1977), while others present the infant responses as two- or three-component waveforms that are only crude approximations of the adult responses (Salamy and McKean, 1976; Schulman-Galambos and Galambos, 1975). A major difference in stimulus protocol

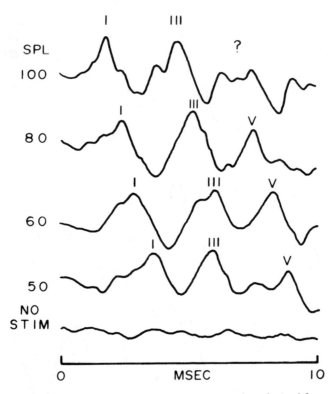

Figure 7.5.   ABRs obtained from an infant. The responses were obtained from a normal-term infant at the age of 17 days.

seems to accompany this difference: the reports of adultlike responses obtained from infants were studies in which the stimulus (click) was presented at a low repetition rate (5 or 10 per second), whereas the other investigations used relatively high stimulus repetition rates (e.g., 30 per second). There appear to be no published investigations of groups of neonatal subjects involving stimulus repetition rates below 10 per second, although some investigators have resorted to low rates occasionally to enhance the detection of the responses (Cox, Hack, and Metz, 1981).

Few reports contain information that would allow an examiner to estimate the probability of detecting each of the various response components in the normal-term infant. There appears to be general agreement that the designated wave V is sufficiently robust to be used as a threshold indicator. Hecox (1975) reports that "there is a great deal of ambiguity associated with picking the peak of wave I" from recordings obtained in very young individuals. He noted that only about 25 to 30% of this group of subjects had a reliable wave I for stimuli presented at

60 dB re: normal adult thresholds. By contrast, Salamy and McKean (1976) report a wave I detection rate of 100% for a group of 90 neonates tested with clicks at 55 dB re: normal adult thresholds. Salamy and McKean also report that wave III was detected in only about 68% of the neonates from whom wave I and wave V measures were obtained. Salamy, McKean, and Buda (1975) noted that waves I and II often merge, and Salamy and McKean (1976) report detection of wave II and wave IV in only 60% and 40% of the neonates, respectively. An impression that emerges from the published data is that one might expect neonates to provide a designated I and V reliably, but that intermediate peaks will be less obvious, even for moderate- and high-intensity stimuli.

The latency of the neonatal response is prolonged when compared with responses obtained from adults for similar stimulus intensities. The amount of latency prolongation decreases very rapidly during the first few weeks of life for infants born prior to 40 weeks gestational age. Schulman-Galambos and Galambos (1975) report a shift of the wave V latency from a mean of 8.57 to 7.3 msec for small groups of infants whose ages were 32 to 42 weeks, and who were stimulated with clicks at 60 dB re: adult thresholds. Starr et al. (1977) report somewhat shorter latencies, but a similar progression for stimuli at 65 dB re: adult thresholds. Starr and coworkers also noted responses from a total of seven infants whose conceptional ages ranged from 26 to 32 weeks. The designated wave V in the youngest infants ranged to 9, 10, or 11 msec in three cases.

Hecox (1975) reports wave V latencies of 7.6 to 8 msec in term infants tested with stimuli at 60 dB re: adult norms. The response latencies decrease to about 6 msec by the 12- to 18-month age range, according to Hecox. Salamy and McKean (1976) report a 7-msec wave V latency for newborns, with a progression to 5.9 msec by 12 months, using clicks at 55 dB re: adult norms. The approximately 6-msec latency noted by Salamy and McKean for 1-year-old children agrees well with the adult latencies summarized in Table 7.1, but within their own populations, Salamy and his coworkers have noted a continual progression of latency through about 32 months.

The interwave intervals determined for neonates are also prolonged when compared with adult values. Salamy and McKean (1976) report an average I–V interval of 5.12 msec for their neonatal population, while their normal adult value is 3.9 msec. Gafni et al. (1980) report a I–V interval of 5.86 msec for neonates tested at 75 dB re: normal adult thresholds. Starr et al. (1977) noted I–V intervals of more than 6 msec for 32-week conceptional-age babies. Their two subjects in the 26- to 28-week age range had I–V intervals of more than 7 msec. This lengthening of the I–V interval reflects the fact that the changes of the absolute latencies of peaks I and V do not progress in a parallel fashion. Generally, it has been observed that the first wave in the normal infant response is delayed only slightly relative to adult values (0.4 msec according to Salamy and McKean, 1976).

A few studies (Hecox and Galambos, 1974; Schulman-Galambos and Galambos, 1975; Mokotoff, Schulman-Galambos, and Galambos, 1977) have provided tabular or graphical representation of the change in neonatal response latency with changes in stimulus intensity. Generally, the response-latency/stimulus-intensity curves of the neonates parallel those of adults, so that a delay noted for high-intensity stimulation is preserved for reductions of stimulus intensity to near-threshold values.

The minimum level of the stimulus for which the infant ABR can be detected has not been reported systematically in the literature. Hecox and Galambos (1974) report testing 35 infants, apparently successfully, with stimuli at 20 dB re: normal adult thresholds. Schulman-Galambos and Galambos (1975) report that all six of their 40- to 42-week gestational-age infants presented responses to stimuli at 30 dB re: adult norms. Hecox (1975) states that the average minimum intensity necessary to obtain the response from newborns was 27 dB re: adult perceptual thresholds. Starr et al. (1977) report using a 25- to 65-dB nHL intensity series, but provide no information on thresholds for their term infants. Schulman-Galambos and Galambos (1975) report responses for 26 of 30 infants tested at 20 dB re: adult perceptual thresholds. This represents only a 10-dB increase over the typical adult ABR *threshold* value reported by their group.

The probability of seeing the ABR for low- and moderate-level stimuli appears to decrease for premature infants. For example, Schulman-Galambos and Galambos (1975) report that only one of six of their 34-week infants responded to stimulation at 30 dB nHL, although all six infants responded to the 60-dB stimulus. Starr et al. (1977) did not observe responses to clicks at 65 dB nHL in the case of one 26-week-old individual. They did note that this individual provided a response at 75 dB, and, interestingly, that a slow cortical response could be obtained from that individual for the 65 dB nHL stimulus, in the absence of the ABR.

At the other end of the age range, Beagley and Sheldrake (1978) have reported on the progression of response latencies for moderate- and high-intensity clicks. Subjects were grouped according to decades of age spanning the range of 11 through 79 years. There were 10 subjects per group, and all individuals were described as having normal hearing, with the exception of a "modest sensorineural loss in the high frequencies" for some of the older subjects. There were no appreciable changes of latency noted with increased age. Rowe (1978) claims to have detected significant shifts of latency for his older subjects, but he failed to test their hearing. Rowe does report that the older subjects' perceptual thresholds for the click stimuli were within 12 dB of the young subjects, but this criterion hardly insures normal or even near normal high-frequency hearing. More recently, Rosenhamer, Lindstrom, and Lundborg (1980) have failed to find significant differences of response latency when responses from persons in the sixth to seventh decade were compared with those from young adults.

Overall, the data related to changes in response characteristics with age suggest that a single set of response threshold and latency norms may be applicable to individuals from the third year of life through the sixth or seventh decade without significant adjustment. Adjustments favoring increased response latencies are essential for the newborn population. It is not certain that an adjustment must be made for the geriatric population if the hearing sensitivity of members of that population is considered along with the ABR results.

Gender The Beagley and Sheldrake (1978) and Rosenhamer, Lindstrom, and Lundborg (1980) studies also examined the effects of subject gender on the characteristics of the response. Beagley and Sheldrake reported that responses obtained from females had shorter latencies that those obtained from males, although the reverse was found for three subjects and there were no differences for five subject pairs. Their impression was that the differences were significant only in a statistical sense. Rosenhamer and coworkers found complex interactions between age and sex, including significant differences between young and old females, but not between the young and old males. They also found shorter latencies for females than for males under the age of 50 years. Michalewski et al. (1980) also note briefer response latencies for females than for males. The differences are in the range of 200 μsec or less. These same three studies also found that responses from female subjects tend to be larger than those from males.

Body Temperature and Drugs The ABR has been shown to be resistant to such factors as attention, sleep state, and a variety of drugs. Stockard, Sharbrough, and Tinker (1978) note, however, that one important sequel to coma and drug intoxication, hypothermia, may influence the latencies of the individual components of the ABR differentially. They report on six cases, five of whom were undergoing coronary surgery. At the lowest body temperature reached by patients during cardiopulmonary bypass (about 8° C below normal body temperature), the I–III intervals were prolonged about 0.7 msec and the III–V intervals were increased by about 0.9 msec over the normal values for the high-intensity clicks used to evaluate the patients. As a result, the I–V intervals were prolonged from their normal value of 3.9 to about 5.5 msec. This was accompanied by a delay of about 0.7 msec for the wave I latency. These findings have obvious importance for applications of the ABR technique during surgery and in intensive-care facilities.

With regard to specific anesthesia effects, Goff et al. (1977) noted minimal (10 to 20%) ABR changes to be associated with the induction of sodium thiopental anesthesia. They did not quantify measures of waves VI and VII but stated that their impression was that those waves were affected more by the anesthesia than were waves I through V. Similar negligible effects have been noted for the earliest components of the ABR in laboratory animals (Bobbin, May, and Lemoine, 1979). A recent study by Javel et al. (1982) suggests that systemic administration of lidocaine hydrochloride results in a prolongation of peak response latencies in cat. The ABR response waveform also was altered in some instances. Lidocaine normally is used as a local anesthetic, but its systemic administration is useful in the stabilization of cardiac rhythm, pain relief, and vestibular symptoms. Therefore, the Javel et al. study would seem to bear repeating in human subjects.

SUMMARY

The ABR is a series of small fluctuations of voltage with latency characteristics that are stable in the normal-hearing and neurologically intact population. The amplitudes of the various components of the ABR are, by contrast, quite variable within and across individual subjects. Generally, the designated wave V of the ABR has been found to be the most robust component. It is also the least susceptible to changes in stimulus repetition rate.

The threshold of the ABR, as determined by the minimum stimulus intensity necessary to elicit a wave V, is within 10 to 20 dB of a normal individual's perceptual threshold for the click stimulus. The earliest portions of the ABR tend to appear when the stimulus reaches moderate suprathreshold levels. The intervals among the peaks elicited by suprathreshold click stimuli remain nearly constant while the entire complex changes latency in an orderly fashion with increases of stimulus intensity.

Some adjustment of normal criteria (latency, amplitude, threshold) is required when one alters stimulation and recording methods or examines very young individuals. Amplitude ratios and latency measures are affected by stimulus rate and filter settings. Threshold measures, response latency, and response waveform undergo dramatic changes during the early days and weeks of life. Overall, however, the response exhibits remarkable stability, and it has been widely accepted as an important supplement to audiometric and neurologic evaluations. Several clinical applications of the ABR technique will be reviewed in the next chapter.

8

CLINICAL APPLICATIONS OF AUDITORY BRAINSTEM RESPONSES

ABR measures have been applied to a broad range of audiological, neurological, and neurosurgical problems. The ABR has been proposed as an indicator of hearing sensitivity in the very young or otherwise difficult-to-test patient, as a means of identifying both discrete and diffuse neurological lesions, and as a method of monitoring the progress of neurosurgical procedures. The ABR results most relevant to audiometric estimation are the response (Wave V) threshold and the relation between latency and stimulus intensity. The neurologic inferences from ABR results are based on measures of interpeak intervals and the relative amplitudes of the various response components. The task of specifying a patient's audiometric status may be compromised if that individual's neurologic status is not normal, and the effects of hearing loss on the ABR may obscure its sensitivity to subtle neurological problems. This chapter will review the effects of hearing loss and neurological problems on the threshold, latency, and morphological characteristics of the ABR.

EFFECTS OF HEARING LOSS ON THE ABR

Threshold Measures   The threshold of the ABR, determined as the detection level for wave V, follows the pattern reviewed in Chapter 6 for the whole nerve AP response. The threshold for click stimuli corresponds roughly to mid- and high-frequency audiometric results and is insensitive to hearing loss confined to the low-frequency region. Jerger and Mauldin (1978) investigated the interaction between extent and configuration of hearing loss and the ABR threshold for a transient stimulus formed by leading one half cycle of a 3,000-Hz sinusoid to conventional earphones. They investigated 275 ears for which audiometric information had been obtained, and found that the ABR threshold correlated best (r = 0.49) with the 4,000-Hz audiometric threshold and the average hearing loss at 1,000, 2,000, and 4,000 Hz (r = 0.48). As Jerger and Mauldin point out, the basic correlation results were not particularly strong and were accompanied by standard deviations in the range of 15 dB. Assuming that behavioral results would be distributed normally about a value estimated by the ABR threshold, this means that the ABR threshold carries with it potentially significant (30-dB) errors with respect to estimation of the audiogram, even in the high-frequency range. Considering the effects of slope of loss and various amounts of average loss, Jerger and Mauldin concluded that the ABR threshold tended to overestimate hearing loss, and that the average threshold for 1, 2, and 4 kHz was best predicted by multiplying the ABR threshold by 0.6.

The uncertainty regarding a prediction from ABR to audiometric results appears to be reduced to perhaps 15 dB as the audiometric configuration flattens in sensorineural (Moller and Blegvad, 1976) or conductive loss (Yamada et al., 1975).

Attempts to improve the audiometric resolution of ABR-based measurements have paralleled the efforts based on the whole nerve AP response (see Chapter 6). There is fair to good agreement between ABR thresholds obtained by using tone bursts or pips and behavioral results in the 2,000 to 8,000 Hz region (cf. Mitchell and Clemis, 1977). The derived response technique has been applied by Don, Eggermont, and Brackmann (1979) to a few patients with excellent results. As they note, however, the technique is time-consuming and probably impractical for routine use. An interesting combination of methods has been reported by Picton et al. (1979). They used brief tonal stimuli presented simultaneously with masking noise. The masking noise was constructed to compete with frequencies beginning one octave above and one octave below the stimulus, with the stimulus frequency corresponding to the "notch" in the noise spectrum. This technique improved predictions of threshold over the use of tone bursts without noise, but appears to be unsatisfactory for low-frequency threshold estimation.

Davis and Hirsh (1979) have suggested that the SN-10 response, which was identified earlier by Suzuki, Hirai, and Horiuchi (1977), may be a reliable indicator of low-frequency (500 Hz) hearing sensitivity in young children. The filter settings and time base used to detect the SN-10 response are different from those employed in conventional ABR procedures. The filter settings used by Davis and Hirsh were 40 to 3,000 Hz, and the time period was extended to 25 msec. They report that the SN-10 appeared as a satisfactory threshold indicator at both 500 and 1,000 Hz. They based their conclusion on the correspondence between the low-frequency SN-10 thresholds and the standard ABR thresholds to higher frequency stimuli. Hawes and Greenberg (1981) report difficulty reproducing the Davis and Hirsh findings, perhaps due to procedural differences involving the filter limits. They did find good correspondence with the Davis and Hirsh conclusions for 1,000 Hz, but not for 500 Hz. Additional observations of Battmer and Lehnhardt (1981) generally were supportive of the Davis and Hirsh findings. Clearly, further exploration of the characteristics of the SN-10 response in normal and hearing-impaired persons is warranted.

In summary, the audiometric inferences that may be drawn from ABR threshold measurements are limited by the same constraints that apply to measures of the AP response. Normal thresholds for click or abrupt tonal stimuli (2 to 8 kHz) appear to predict normal hearing in the mid- and high-frequency region in a satisfactory manner. When one encounters a significant ABR threshold shift (in the absence of a retro-cochlear disorder) it is probable that a hearing loss is present in the high-frequency region. However, estimates of the audiogram shape are very tenuous if one considers only the ABR threshold results or any other measure based on a single stimulus intensity. Consideration of the response latency with changes in stimulus intensity will sometimes help to clarify the audiometric picture.

ABR Latency-Intensity Measurements   Figure 8.1 is an illustration of the latency of wave V for a group of normal subjects and for two individuals with hearing loss. Generally, conductive hearing loss involving the high-frequency region will produce a shift in the response latency/stimulus-intensity function to the right on the intensity axis, but the general slope of the function will be normal. Sensorineural hearing loss due to cochlear disorders often results in a steep latency/intensity function, with the wave V latency approaching near-normal values for high-intensity stimuli (cf. Galambos and Hecox, 1977; Picton et al., 1977; Skinner and Glattke, 1977; Yamada, Kodera, and Yagi, 1979).

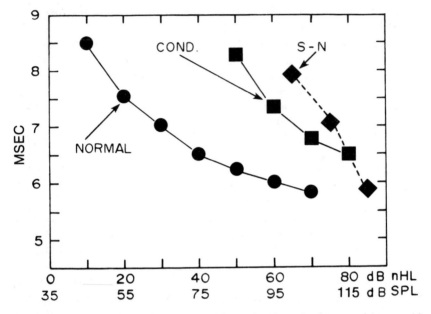

Figure 8.1.   Examples of latency measures obtained in normal subjects and in two with conductive and sensorineural (S-N) hearing loss. Both patients experienced an average loss of approximately 45 to 50 dB through the high-frequency range.

The prolongation of the latency of wave V associated with conductive hearing loss can also be found in two other conditions: precipitous high-frequency hearing loss and the presence of a space-occupying lesion affecting the auditory nerve. For example, Yamada, Kodera, and Yagi (1979) noted that patients with high-frequency hearing loss who reveal only a slight to mild elevation of ABR wave V threshold may exhibit response latencies that fail to reach the normal latency range of wave V. The resulting prolongation of latency at high stimulus intensities was to more than 1 msec in one instance reported by Yamada, Kodera, and Yagi. Coats (1978) reports a systematic increase in wave V latency as the extent of hearing loss in the 4,000 to 8,000 region increases, but refrained from specifying mean and standard deviations because of the small number of subjects in each of his groups.

While the specific effects of space-occupying lesions will be discussed in a later section of this chapter, it should be noted that Selters and Brackmann (1977, 1979) have reported that a simple determination of the *interaural latency difference* (ILD) of wave V has great sensitivity for the presence of a tumor involving the auditory nerve. Using high-intensity stimuli, they noted that latency differences between the good and suspect ear that were greater than 0.2 msec were common to many patients with confirmed tumors. They suggested correcting for hearing loss at 4 kHz by reducing the measured delay in the suspect ear by 0.1 msec for each 10-dB increment of hearing loss above 50 dB HL. The correction is required to prevent persons with hearing loss not due to tumors from being categorized as possible tumor patients on the basis of the wave V ILD criterion. Rosenhamer, Lindstrom, and Lundborg (1981a, 1981b) found a correction of 0.1 msec per 10-dB loss beginning at 30 dB was appropriate for their pool of subjects.

Many clinical examiners tend to favor use of a single high-intensity stimulus to gather ABRs for the purpose of assessment of response latency and other characteristics. Therefore, it is appropriate to consider the possible effects of hearing loss on responses obtained for high-intensity stimulation. In addition to the four studies cited above, recent work includes that of Rosenhamer, Lindstrom, and Lundborg (1981a), who investigated 110 patients with click stimuli at 80 dB nHL. Patients were grouped according to amount of hearing loss at 4 kHz. Increases in the latency of wave V were noted to vary directly with the amount of loss. The mean increase for patients with mild (30- to 35-dB) loss was 0.14 msec. This grew to 0.6 msec for individuals with hearing loss exceeding 90 dB. The standard deviation of latencies for wave V for the most severe hearing loss group was 0.3 msec. Sohmer, Kinarti, and Gafni (1981) also investigated this question using a small group of patients with sensorineural hearing loss. They report an average 0.35 msec increase in the latency of wave V at 75 dB nHL.

Taken together, data regarding the effects of hearing loss on the intensity/latency characteristics of wave V suggest that hearing loss in the peripheral auditory system will prolong the latency of wave V. The amount of prolongation depends on the amount of hearing loss in the high-frequency region, and it follows that the interpretation of ABRs with respect to latency will be enhanced with information about audiometric status. Determining audiometric status solely on the basis of ABR results is difficult. The existence of a hearing loss that includes the high-frequency region usually can be demonstrated through ABR threshold measures. A steep latency/intensity function suggests a cochlear disorder and may reflect a hearing loss confined to the high-frequency region. A latency function for wave V that is prolonged and parallels the normal curve raises several possibilities that must be explored before a final diagnosis can be reached. Ruling out significant conductive hearing loss is straightforward in this instance, but separation of cochlear and retrocochlear disorders may be impossible.

Hearing Loss and Interwave Interval Measurements   It generally is held that the latency of wave I is dictated by the external and the middle ear and by cochlear responses. The intervals between wave I and subsequent waves and the intervals among the later waves are thought to be determined by the status of the auditory nerve and central nervous system. Therefore, if one wishes to use measurements of the ABR as an aid to neurologic diagnosis, the interwave interval measurements assume primary importance. A fundamental question that must be answered relates to the effect of peripheral hearing loss on the interwave interval characteristics.

Review of the data summarized in Table 7.2 suggests that the interwave intervals associated with click stimuli are reduced slightly as the intensity of the stimulus decreases toward response threshold in normal listeners. The decrease is most apparent for the I–III interval and is echoed as a I–V interval decrease. Results similar to those summarized in Table 7.2 were reported by Stockard et al. (1979) for stimuli ranging from 30 through 70 dB SL. Their findings suggested that the I–V interval change did not simply mirror the I–III change, however. They reported an average 0.19 msec I–III reduction, and a 0.34 msec I–V interval reduction as the stimuli were reduced to 30 dB SL. More complete latency-intensity studies reported by Coats (1978) also suggest a systematic abbreviation of the intervals between the whole nerve AP response (presumed to be wave I in the ABR) and wave V as hearing loss increases in the high-frequency region. Whereas the normal I–V interval is approximately 4 msec for stimuli of moderate intensity in normal individuals, Coats found the interval to decrease to less than 3.5 msec for *near-threshold stimulation of persons with moderate to severe hearing loss.* The intervals returned to normal values when responses were obtained for stimuli 30 to 40 dB above the ABR threshold values.

The decrease of the interwave intervals generally can be traced to the fact that the latency of the designated wave I shifts to a greater extent than the latency of the later waves. As a result, there is an abbreviation of the interval between the first *detected* wave and wave V. This poses a dilemma for the clinician who must compare data from a specific patient to normal data, especially if the clinician prefers to use only a single stimulus intensity for the purpose of obtaining ABRs. For example, if the clinical evaluation uses a stimulus presented at 80 dB nHL, and the ABR threshold of the patient is not known, then the examiner will not know whether to expect abbreviated or "normal" I–V intervals. Once again, the importance of obtaining audiometric information and a series of ABR measurements at several stimulus intensities is self-evident.

EFFECTS OF RETROCOCHLEAR DISORDERS ON THE ABR

The broad category of retrocochlear disorders includes space-occupying lesions, degenerative disorders, or those secondary to malformation or trauma. As Fria (1980) has asserted, the available evidence does not permit us to identify ABR characteristics peculiar to any specific disease entity. Rather, ABR findings permit initial categorization of patient anomalies into broad "peripheral" or "central" categories where the break-point between the two categories appears to be the internal auditory meatus. Generally, abnormalities of the peripheral apparatus, including the cochlea and distal part of the auditory nerve, are reflected in response alterations that can be traced back to the characteristics of the auditory nerve response. Aberrations of the response beyond wave I are associated with the medial portion of the auditory nerve and the central nervous system. The changes in the ABR that are of most interest from the neurological standpoint are (1) interwave interval measures and (2) changes in response waveform caused by other than simple shifts of latency.

Lesions Involving the Auditory Nerve   Space-occupying lesions involving the auditory nerve directly are manifested by aberrations of both response waveform and interpeak intervals. Eggermont, Don, and Brackmann (1980) report a failure to detect wave V in 15 of 43 (35%) patients with acoustic nerve tumors. Selters and Brackmann (1977) failed to record wave V in 54% of a group of 46 patients with tumors. Rosenhamer (1977) failed to obtain ABRs in all of 13 cases with large (>2-cm) tumors. Eleven of those 13 patients had normal ABRs on stimulation of the ear contralateral to the tumor, and two revealed "partially normal" responses for contralateral stimulation. The ABR results with contralateral abnormalities were thought to be associated with dislocation of the brainstem. Twelve patients with medium-size tumors (1- to 2-cm) in Rosenhamer's group failed to produce an ABR "that was reproducible to 30 dB SL stimulation." Among five patients with smaller tumors, the responses were present, but abnormal. Clemis and McGee (1979) report failure to detect ABRs in 16% of 26 patients having relatively small (<1-cm) tumors. Collectively, reports that have included information about the probability of detection of ABRs in cases of tumors involving the auditory nerve suggest that the size of the tumor directly affects the examiner's ability to detect a repeatable response.

A natural consequence of increases of interwave intervals is the prolongation of wave V latency, and, as mentioned earlier, Selters and Brackmann (1977) and others noted that a comparison of wave V latencies may help to detect unilateral tumors. Clemis and McGee (1979) confirmed that the ILD offers great sensitivity to tumors, with a 93% detection rate. They also demonstrated, however, that ILD measurement is not a very precise indicator of the presence of tumors. They report a 37% false positive indication of tumors among 128 nontumor patients when using absolute wave V latency measurements or ILD comparisons. Thirteen of these 128 patients had conductive loss, and an abnormal ILD or missing wave V was reported for all of those patients. The remaining false positives were distributed among various patients with sensorineural hearing loss. Bauch, Rose, and Harner (1982) report a similar experience with 255 patients (25% false positive ABR results).

Clemis and McGee (1979) report that two of 26 persons with confirmed tumors presented false negative results using the absolute wave V latency or ILD criteria. Eggermont, Don, and Brackmann (1980) report a similar false negative rate using the ILD criterion. Coats (1978) reported a 21.4% false negative rate when absolute wave V latency measures obtained from tumor patients were compared with the results obtained from other patients having sensorineural hearing loss. This was reduced to a 14% false negative rate when the measurements for tumor patients were contrasted with the results from normal-hearing individuals, but the reduction of false negatives was accompanied by an increase in false positives from 0 to 13.5%.

Coats (1978), Eggermont, Don, and Brackmann (1980), and Portmann et al. (1980) have presented strong arguments for focusing on measures of the I–V interval, rather than absolute wave V latencies or ILD. These authors note that *combined* cochleographic (with ear-canal or promontory electrodes) and ABR recordings can remove many of the uncertainties associated with total reliance on ABR when wave I cannot be identified in the ABR recording. Examples of response latencies illustrated in Figure 8.2 reveal how the uncertainty can be resolved. Each panel consists of a plot of response latencies and I–V intervals for a specific patient. The results from the individual patient may be contrasted with the normal range illustrated by the smooth curvilinear lines. The results from the cochlear patient are associated with precipitous high-frequency hearing loss. As a consequence of the loss, the latency measures are prolonged for both wave V and wave I. The interval measurement is entirely normal for all stimuli. The results illustrated in the case of retrocochlear lesions are distinct in that the I–V intervals are prolonged consistently for all stimuli. The case illustrated in panel B reveals a prolongation or wave I and a greater prolongation of wave V. Hence, the interwave intervals exceed 5 msec. The results summarized in panel C include a normal wave I characteristic and an isolated prolongation of wave V. When the I–V intervals were considered by Coats (1978), the false positive rate fell to 0% and the false negative rate was 7 to 14% for detection of retrocochlear lesions. Coats's determination of abnormality included a requirement that 50% of the data points on the interwave-interval/stimulus-intensity curves were outside of the normal range. He noted that an earlier study (Coats and Martin, 1977) produced

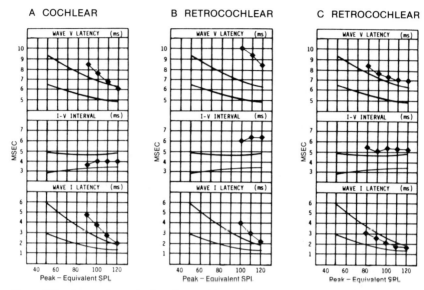

Figure 8.2.   Latency/intensity functions and interval measure in cochlear and retrocochlear hearing loss.

a 5% false positive rate when only single-intensity measures were obtained.

Relying solely on surface-recorded ABRs, Eggermont, Don, and Brackmann (1980) specified a 4.1-msec average interval between waves I and V for clicks at 70 dB nHL. Because the standard deviation associated with this mean was 0.16 msec, they employed a maximum I–V interval limit of 4.49 msec (+3 standard deviations) to separate probable tumor from nontumor patients. Among 28 patients for whom wave V could be recorded, 24 revealed prolonged I–V intervals, two were borderline normal, and two were within normal limits. This represents a detection rate of about 86%, a false negative rate of 7% and a 7% incidence of questionable results. When they employed their ILD criterion, the two patients who were classified as questionable moved clearly into the abnormal category. Their study did not include consideration of nontumor patients, and false positives could not be reported.

As Eggermont, Don, and Brackmann noted, cochleographic procedures supply additional information when results indicate a tumor and the ABR results are normal. One of their two patients with false negative findings with ABR presented abnormal AP findings. Portmann et al. (1980) report reliance on cochleographic procedures to obtain their I–V interval measures for patients having retrocochlear disorders and hearing loss in excess of 40 dB, because no wave I could be detected from surface electrodes in those instances. They employed a 4.5 msec I–V interval limit for purposes of separation of their cochlear and retro-cochlear patients, and had a false negative rate of 7%. They also mis-classified one of 26 (4%) of the cochlear patients into their retrocochlear category on the basis of prolonged interval measurements.

Overall, the various studies that have examined ABR and electro-cochleographic correlates to the presence of space-occupying lesions in-volving the auditory nerve suggest that the combination of ILD and I–V interval measurements will result in detection of a tumor in more than 85% of the cases. The detection rate rises when one also considers un-measurable (absent) ABRs, especially where there is little or no hearing loss. Eggermont, Don, and Brackmann (1980) stated that their overall 95% detection rate "must be regarded as optimum. It is not likely to occur in the real diagnostic situation in which one does not know if a pontine angle tumor is present." Thus, consideration of the ABR results in the context of other audiological information remains important to the diagnostic process (Jerger, Neely, and Jerger, 1980).

Nonauditory Nerve Tumors   Tumors involving the brainstem or midbrain structures while sparing the auditory nerve produce response abnormalities that correlate only in a general sense with the focus of the lesion. Stockard, Stockard, and Sharbrough (1977) report an increase in the III-V interval for an astrocytoma involving the caudal brainstem and extending superficially to the junction of the pons and medulla. A caudal pontine glioma was associated with reduction of the amplitude of waves III and V. Starr and Hamilton (1976) report a case involving a neoplasm that invaded the midbrain and upper pons. The ABRs presented with this case reveal obliteration of the response components beyond wave III. Jerger, Neely, and Jerger (1980) report an instance of a primary tumor in the midbrain with ABRs that were normal through wave V. Stockard and Rossiter (1977) report a normal latency of wave V for a case involving a pineal body tumor, but they and others (Hashimoto, Ishiyama, and Tozuka, 1979) also report increases in the III–V interval for midbrain lesions. Abnormalities of both amplitude and latency have also been noted. For example, Lynn et al. (1981) report III–V interval increases and V amplitude reduction for a person with a pineal body tumor.

Diffuse Lesion Effects   Diffuse lesions appear to be related to a variety of ABR patterns. Reporting on patients who were classified as meeting the criteria for brain death, Starr (1976) noted that wave I was the only ABR component that could be recorded in about 40% of a group of 27 patients. The other patients produced no responses. In one interesting case that was followed during the period when the patient's condition deteriorated, the amplitude of wave I increased, possibly reflecting disinhibition of the auditory nerve response. Black et al. (1979) and Ochs, Markland, and DeMyer (1979) have reported both interval increases and loss of response components beyond wave I in patients with leukodystrophy. One of the Ochs group's cases, involving suspected early adrenoleukodystrophy, revealed normal standard EEG findings and a selective prolongation of the interval between waves IV and V.

Patients with multiple sclerosis have been studied with ABR techniques by several authors. Stockard, Stockard, and Sharbrough (1977) report on a series of 100 patients, and stated that 93% of 30 patients with a "definite" diagnosis of MS had ABR abnormalities. These included abnormalities of amplitude, latency, or both in approximately even distributions across the subject pool. Among 30 "probable" MS patients, 77% had abnormal ABRs. Thirty-five percent of 40 "possible" MS patients revealed ABR abnormalities. Stephens and Thornton (1976) report on 10 MS patients among a group of 22 with disorders of the brainstem and noted that latency prolongations without amplitude changes were the most common observations in the MS group. Robinson and Rudge (1977) report that 63% of 51 MS patients had abnormalities of wave V amplitude or latency. They also used a paired-click paradigm in which responses were examined for double clicks separated by 5 msec, and noted that three patients who had previously revealed normal responses to single clicks (presented with an interval of 50 msec) had abnormal responses to the second member of the click pair. Mogensen and Kristensen (1979) report a small increase in the detection of abnormalities of the ABR among MS patients when double clicks separated by 5 msec were used.

Overall, the reports about patients with multiple sclerosis suggest that there will be ABR abnormalities in a high proportion of selected patients, but that there is no clear pattern of ABR associated with the disorder. Some of the discrepant results reported for MS patients may be understood by a consideration of the work of Parving, Elberling, and Smith (1981), who examined 15 patients having a definite diagnosis of MS. Their evaluations included electrocochleographic studies in some cases, and they noted subtle changes in the AP amplitude/latency functions in the midintensity range. Thirteen of their patients were evaluated using ABR techniques at three intensities ranging from 65 through 85 dB nHL. They assembled "average responses" of their patients by summing across patient records, and identified two subgroups within their sample. No clear wave V latency increase was observed in any patient, and seven of the 13 patients revealed no gross morphological changes in the ABR. However, the remaining six patients presented

ABRs that consisted of a combination of small waves with a relatively large and slow voltage shift. The shift reached its maximum amplitude at a moment coincident with wave V for high stimulus levels, but was prolonged (to 8 or 10 msec) for the 65-dB nHL stimulus. This sustained slow component, coexisting with smaller fast waves, can obscure the fast waves. If the largest response peak is always designated as wave V, the slow component can be confused with the true wave V. An important practical implication of this study is that wave V may be misidentified if one always identifies it as the largest response component in the time period exceeding 5.5 msec. Their summary suggests "a strong need for applying . . . objective methods of analysis to identify and evaluate the various components of the evoked potentials." As their careful analysis revealed no true abnormalities of the wave V latency, their findings echo the observations of Achor and Starr (1980b), who found no latency shifts due to discrete lesions placed in laboratory animals.

SPECIAL PROBLEMS AND POPULATIONS

Undetected Unilateral Deafness   ABRs obtained from a patient with undetected unilateral deafness may be subject to misinterpretation because of cross-over of the acoustic stimulus to the better ear. In the worst case, where one ear is normal and the other is not functioning, stimuli delivered to the deaf ear by conventional earphones may be detected in the better ear when they reach approximately 50 to 60 dB nHL. Thus, if the examiner stimulates the deaf ear at 80 dB nHL, a near-threshold ABR will be detected because of the contribution of the normal ear. This response, due to stimulation of the better ear at 20 to 30 dB SL, will consist of a prolonged wave V, with a latency in the range of 7 to 8 msec. In essence, the response from the good ear resembles that associated with a *conductive hearing loss*. In this case the conductive loss is produced by the attenuation of the headphone cushions and skull in the process of transmitting the stimulus to the nontest ear. Should an ABR examination reveal normal responses from one ear (including normal thresholds) and significant threshold elevation for the other ear, reevaluation of the poor ear should be conducted with masking noise in the normal ear. Elimination of the response with masking in the normal, nontest ear will confirm the presence of a cross-over effect.

Multiply Handicapped Patients   One popular use of the ABR is in the area of evaluating the hearing of difficult-to-test patients. The audiometric limitations posed by the use of transient stimuli have been discussed elsewhere in this book. If normal thresholds and latencies are found for an individual, the examiner may interpret those findings to mean that the patient probably has normal high-frequency hearing sensitivity. If the responses are absent or reveal significant elevation of threshold, the interpretation must be guarded. This is because the neurological status of the patient, rather than hearing sensitivity, may affect the response (Squires et al., 1980). The report of Worthington and Peters (1980b) illustrates this dilemma. They found an absence of repeatable ABRs in approximately 1% of a large population of children referred because of speech or language disorders. The patients exhibited various degrees of hearing loss, but none were deaf. Ryerson and Beagley (1981) evaluated 46 children using both cochleographic and ABR procedures and concluded that reliance on ABR measures alone could be misleading. They observed that normal thresholds by ABR could be confirmed easily by cochleographic techniques. They also found that the cochleography results indicated much lower thresholds than the ABR in about 10% of their patients. Ryerson and Beagley recommend that cochleographic procedures be added to the assessment protocol if the ABR thresholds are elevated by more than 30 dB nHL. As neither the cochleographic nor the ABR techniques are true tests of "hearing" it is mandatory that their interpretation be couched in the context of other findings, including tympanometric studies, behavioral observations, and assessment of the overall developmental characteristics of the person undergoing evaluation.

Evaluation of Neonatal Hearing   The neonatal population poses special problems because of the interaction of normal maturation, hearing sensitivity, and possible undetected neurological disorders on the ABR. The studies of developmental aspects of the ABR cited previously suggest the technique as sensitive to all three factors, but often it is difficult to determine the specific cause of the absence of a response in the neonate. As a result, widely varying estimates of the prevalence of neonatal hearing loss have appeared in the literature. For example, Despland and Galambos (1980) evaluated 91 premature infants and reached conclusions regarding neurologic and audiologic status by using ABR threshold, latency, and interwave interval measurements. They stated that 11 (12%) of the 91 patients gave evidence of a hearing disorder. No followup audiological data were available and so it is not possible to determine how many of those patients actually had a significant hearing loss. The followup data are important because graduates of neonatal intensive-care units frequently reveal recovery of the ABR within a few weeks or months after leaving the hospital. For example Roberts et al. (1982) reported that 36 of 75 (48%) neonatal intensive-care patients failed a screening procedure requiring a response to be present at

40 dB nHL. On followup, only one case of significant hearing loss (1.3%) was confirmed. Galambos, Hicks, and Wilson (1982) found that 141 of 890 (16%) infants who survived after a stay in an intensive-care unit failed screening at 30 dB nHL. Followup was provided for about 43% of those who failed the screening, and only 16 of those persons ultimately were fitted with hearing aids. The Galambos, Hicks, and Wilson (1982) study suggests that approximately 2% of the neonates in the intensive-care nursery will have significant hearing loss (16 of 890). The clinical examiner who offers ABR testing as a routine clinical screening will have to deal with the probability that many patients will fail the screen, only to have a normal result at a later time. In the case of the Galambos, Hicks, and Wilson study, only one of every four children who were followed because of the initial screen ultimately required hearing aids. Roberts et al. (1982) express doubts as to whether the application of ABR screening procedures, even for patients who are at risk for hearing loss, is cost effective. Downs (1982) has criticized the routine screening of neonatal intensive-care infants on the basis of the lack of demonstrated reliability, hence validity, and the relatively sparse normative data. He argues that the high false positive rate and limited information associated with the screening may make the procedure counterproductive.

SUMMARY

The evaluation of the ABR has found widespread application in clinical practice. It has been shown to be a very sensitive indicator of both peripheral and central disorders associated with the auditory system. There is ample evidence that results of the ABR evaluation, like those of most specialized tests, cannot be interpreted in isolation. The ABR cannot be used to measure "hearing." Abnormalities of the response can help to raise the examiner's index of suspicion for the presence of hearing loss or for other problems.

   If a patient's ABR threshold, waveform, and latency-intensity characteristics are normal, then one usually will be able to infer that the individual's pure tone audiometric results will be normal in the high-frequency region. Elevation of the ABR threshold must be interpreted with the same constraint that applies to the analysis of whole nerve AP results. In addition, the examiner must be wary of the possible influence of undetected neurological disorders. This may pose a serious problem in the evaluation of the hearing of multiply handicapped patients. The derived response technique appears to improve the examiner's ability to estimate low-frequency audiometric configurations, and perhaps some type of screening protocol can be developed from it. The SN-10 response also appears to warrant additional study for the purpose of audiogram estimation.

The latency of the ABR, particularly when evaluated over a range of stimulus intensities, carries information about both type of hearing loss and neurological status of the patient. Abnormal latency results require that hearing loss be ruled out (or considered) before arriving at conclusions regarding neurologic status. Generally, the amount of latency prolongation of wave V is directly related to the amount of hearing loss in the high-frequency region.

If wave I can be measured with confidence, the I–V interval can be used to separate the effects of hearing loss and retrocochlear problems. This procedure may be enhanced by simultaneous recording of the isolated AP response and the ABR in some patients. Neurological disorders not manifested by a hearing loss present a variety of ABR findings, including an increase in the latency of wave V, an increase in the intervals among waves, changes in the amplitude of various components, and gross distortions of the response waveform. Tumors involving the auditory nerve are manifested primarily by a delay between wave I and later waves (or a loss of the later portion of the response). Destruction of structures within the brainstem and midbrain correlate in a general way with loss or modification of the various waves in the response. Patients with diffuse lesions evidence a broad range of response abnormalities, including combinations of latency changes and waveform changes.

Table 8.1 provides a brief summary of alternatives that an examiner must consider when confronted with various outcomes of an ABR evaluation. "Retrocochlear involvement" refers to any of a variety of disorders (tumors, degenerative disease, etc.) that may influence the test outcome independently of a loss of hearing.

Table 8.1. Some possible outcomes of ABR measurements

Test outcome	Conclusions/additional questions
Normal threshold and latency characteristics	Normal high-frequency hearing sensitivity
Elevated threshold, normal I–V interval, prolonged absolute latency of V	Probable hearing loss in the high-frequency region without retrocochlear involvement
Elevated threshold, prolonged I–V interval	Probable retrocochlear involvement
Abnormal waveform	Probable retrocochlear involvement Determine if the response is near threshold
No I, poor definition of V	Conductive loss, severe SN loss, or retrocochlear disorder Rule out dead ear

REFERENCES

Achor, L. J., and Starr, A. 1980a. Auditory brain stem responses in the cat. I. Intracranial and extracranial recordings. Electroenceph. Clin. Neurophysiol. 48:154–173.

Achor, L. J., and Starr, A. 1980b. Auditory brain stem responses in the cat. II. Effects of lesion. Electroenceph. Clin. Neurophysiol. 48:174–190.

Antoli-Candela, F., and Kiang, N. Y. S. 1978. Unit activity underlying the N1 potential. In: R. F. Naunton and C. Fernandez (eds.), Evoked Electrical Activity in the Auditory Nervous System, pp. 165–191. Academic Press, New York.

Aran, J.-M. 1971. The electrocochleogram: Recent results in children and in some pathological cases. Arch. Ohr. Nas. Kehlk Heilk. 198:128–141.

Aran, J.-M. and Charlet de Sauvage, R. 1976. Clinical value of cochlear microphonic recordings. In: R. J. Ruben, C. Elberling, and G. Salomon (eds.), Electrocochleography, pp. 55–65. University Park Press, Baltimore.

Aran, J.-M., Charlet de Sauvage, R., and Pelerin, J. 1971. Comparaison des seuils électrocochléographiques et de l'audiogramme. Etude statistique. Rev. Laryngol. Otol. Rhinol. (Bordeaux) 92:477–491.

Battmer, R. D., and Lehnhardt, E. 1981. The brain stem response SN_{10}, its frequency selectivity and its value in classifying neural hearing lesions. Arch. Otorhinolaryngol. 230:37–47.

Bauch, C. D., Rose, D. E., and Harner, S. G. 1982. Auditory brain stem response results from 255 patients with suspected retrocochlear involvement. Ear Hear. 3:83–86.

Beagley, H. A., and Gibson, W. P. R. 1978. Electrocochleography in adults. In: R. F. Naunton and C. Fernandez (eds.), Evoked Electrical Activity in the Auditory Nervous System, pp. 259–273. Academic Press, New York.

Beagley, H. A., and Sheldrake, J. B. 1978. Differences in brainstem response latency with age and sex. Br. J. Audiol. 12:69–77.

Black, J. A., Ruggero, G., Fariello, G., and Chun, R. W. 1979. Brainstem auditory evoked response in adrenoleukodystrophy. Ann. Neurol. 6:269–270.

109

Bobbin, R., May, J. G., and Lemoine, R. L. 1979. Effects of pentobarbital and ketamine on brain stem auditory potentials. Arch. Otolaryngol. 105:467–470.

Brackmann, D. E., and Selters, W. A. 1976. Electrocochleography in Meniere's disease and acoustic neuromas. In: R. J. Ruben, C. Elberling, and G. Salomon (eds.), Electrocochleography, pp. 315–329. University Park Press, Baltimore.

Chiappa, K. H., Gladstone, K. J., and Young, R. R. 1979. Brainstem auditory evoked responses: Studies of waveform variations in 50 normal human subjects. Arch. Neurol. 36:81–87.

Clemis, J. D., and McGee, T. 1979. Brain stem electric response audiometry in the differential diagnosis of acoustic tumors. Laryngoscope 89:31–42.

Coats, A. C. 1974. On electrocochleographic electrode design. J. Acoust. Soc. Am. 56:708–711.

Coats, A. C. 1978. Human auditory nerve action potentials and brain stem evoked responses: Latency-intensity functions in detection of cochlear and retrocochlear abnormality. Arch. Otolaryngol. 104:709–717.

Coats, A. C. 1981. The summating potential and Meniere's disease. I. Summating potential amplitude in Meniere and non-Meniere ears. Arch. Otolaryngol. 107:199–208.

Coats, A. C., and Dickey, J. R. 1970. Nonsurgical recording of human auditory nerve potentials and cochlear microphonics. Ann. Otol. 79:844–852.

Coats, A. C., and Jerger, J. 1979. Auditory Evoked Potentials Course Syllabus. The Neurosensory Center of Houston, Texas.

Coats, A. C., and Kidder, H. R. 1980. Earspeaker coupling effects on auditory action potential and brain stem responses. Arch. Otolaryngol. 106:339–344.

Coats, A. C., and Martin, J. L. 1977. Human auditory nerve action potentials and brain stem evoked responses: Effects of audiogram shape and lesion location. Arch. Otolaryngol. 103:605–622.

Coats, A. C., Martin, J. L., and Kidder, H. R. 1979. Normal short latency electrophysiological filtered click responses from vertex and external auditory meatus. J. Acoust. Soc. Am. 65:747–758.

Cox, C., Hack, M., and Metz, D. 1981. Brainstem evoked response audiometry: Normative data from the preterm infant. Audiology 20:53–64.

Cullen J. K., Ellis, M. S., Berlin, C. I., and Lousteau, R. J. 1972. Human acoustic nerve action potential recordings from the tympanic membrane without anesthesia. Acta Oto-laryng. 74:15–22.

Dallos, P. 1973. The Auditory Periphery. Academic Press, New York.

Davis, H. 1976. Principles of electric response audiometry. Ann. Otol. Suppl. 28:1–96.

Davis, H., and Hirsh, S. K. 1979. A slow brain stem response for low-frequency audiometry. Audiology 18:445–461.

Davis, H., Silverman, S. R., and McAulfie, D. R. 1951. Some observations on pitch and frequency. J. Acoust. Soc. Am. 23:40–42.

Despland, P. A., and Galambos, R. 1980. The auditory brainstem response (ABR) is a useful diagnostic tool in the intensive care nursery. Pediat. Res. 14:154–158.

Don, M., Allen, A. R., and Starr, A. 1977. Effect of click rate on the latency of auditory brain stem responses in humans. Ann. Otol. 86:186–195.

Don, M., and Eggermont, J. J. 1978. Analysis of the click-evoked brainstem potentials in man using high-pass noise masking. J. Acoust. Soc. Am. 63:1084–1092.

Don, M., Eggermont, J. J., and Brackmann, D. E. 1979. Reconstruction of the audiogram using brain stem responses and high-pass noise masking. Ann. Otol. Suppl. 57:1–20.

Downs, D. W. 1982. Auditory brain stem response testing in the neonatal intensive care unit: A cautious perspective. Asha. 24:1009–1015.

Durrant, J. D., and Phillips, C. M. 1979. An AC ohmeter for electrode impedance measurements. J. Acoust. Soc. Am. 65:1065–1066.

Durrant, J. D., and Ronis, M. L. 1975. Remote extracochlea versus intracochlear recordings in the guinea pig. Ann. Otol. 84:88–93.

Eggermont, J. J. 1976a. Electrocochleography. In: W. D. Keidel and W. D. Neff (eds.), Handbook of Sensory Physiology, Vol. V/3, pp. 626–705. Springer-Verlag, New York.

Eggermont, J. J. 1976b. Summating potentials in electrocochleography: Relation to hearing disorders. In: R. J. Ruben, C. Elberling, and G. Salomon (eds.), Electrocochleography, pp. 67–87. University Park Press, Baltimore.

Eggermont, J. J. 1979. Summating potentials in Meniere's disease. Arch. Otorhinolaryngol. 222:63–75.

Eggermont, J. J., and Don, M. 1980. Analysis of the click-evoked brainstem potentials in humans using high-pass noise masking. II. Effect of click intensity. J. Acoust. Soc. Am. 68:1671–1675.

Eggermont, J. J., Don, M., and Brackmann, D. E. 1980. Electrocochleography and auditory brainstem electric responses in patients with pontine angle tumors. Ann. Otol. Suppl. 75:1–19.

Eggermont, J. J., Odenthal, D. W., Schmidt, P. H., and Spoor, A. 1974. Electrocochleography. Basic principles and clinical application. Acta Oto-laryng. Suppl. (Stockholm) 316:1–84.

Eggermont, J. J., Spoor, A., and Odenthal, D. W. 1976. Frequency specificity of tone-burst electrocochleography. In: R. J. Ruben, C. Elberling, and G. Salomon (eds.), Electrocochleography, pp. 215–246. University Park Press, Baltimore.

Elberling, C. 1974. Action potentials along the cochlear partition recorded from the ear canal in man. Scand. Audiol. 3:13–19.

Evans, E. F. 1975. The sharpening of cochlear frequency selectivity in the normal and abnormal cochlea. Audiology 14:419–422.

Fabiani, M., Sohmer, H., Tait, C., Gafni, M., and Kinarti, R. 1979. A functional measure of brain activity: Brain stem transmission time. Electroenceph. Clin. Neurophysiol. 47:483–491.

Fria, T. J. 1980. The auditory brain stem response: Background and clinical applications. Monographs in Contemporary Audiology 2(2):1–44. Maico Hearing Instruments, Minneapolis.

Fujikawa, S., and Weber, B. A. 1977. Effects of increased stimulus rate on brainstem response (BER) audiometry as a function of age. J. Am. Audiol. 3:147–150.

Funasaka, S., and Abe, H. 1979. Cochlear and fast electrical responses to frequency modulated tones: A frequency specific stimulus. Auris. Nasis. Larynx (Tokyo) 6:59–69.

Gafni, M., Sohmer, H., Gross, S., Weizman, Z., and Robinson, M. J. 1980. Analysis of auditory nerve–brainstem responses (ABR) in neonates and very young infants. Arch. Otorhinolaryngol. 229:167–174.

Galambos, R., and Hecox, K. 1977. Clinical applications of the brainstem potentials. In: J. E. Desmedt (ed.), Auditory Evoked Potentials in Man: Psychopharmacology Correlates of Evoked Potentials, pp. 1–19. S. Karger, Basel.

Galambos, R., Hicks, G., and Wilson, M. J. 1982. Hearing loss in graduates of a tertiary intensive care nursery. Ear Hear. 3:87–90.

Gibson, W. P. R. 1978. Essentials of Clinical Evoked Response Audiometry. Churchill Livingstone, New York.

Gibson, W. P. R., and Beagley, H. A. 1976. Transtympanic electrocochleography in the investigation of retro-cochlear disorders. Rev. Laryngol. Otol. Rhinol. Suppl. (Bordeaux) 97:507–516.

Gibson, W. P. R., Moffat, D. A., and Ramsden, R. T. 1977. Clinical electrocochleography in the diagnosis and management of Meniere's disorder. Audiology 16:389–401.

Glattke, T. J. 1972. Human auditory nerve responses in the presence of band-limited noise. Presented at the Convention of the American Speech-Language-Hearing Association, November, San Francisco.

Glattke, T. J. 1976. Short latency evoked responses to amplitude-modulated tones. Presented at the Convention of the American Speech-Language-Hearing Association, November, Houston.

Glattke, T. J. 1978. Electrocochleography. In: J. Katz (ed.), Handbook of Clinical Audiology, 2nd Ed., pp. 328–343. Williams and Wilkins, Baltimore.

Glattke, T. J. 1980. Sound and hearing. In: T. J. Hixon, L. D. Shriberg, and J. H. Saxman (eds.), Introduction to Communication Disorders, pp. 89–135. Prentice-Hall, Inc., Englewood Cliffs, New Jersey.

Goff, W. R., Allison, T., Lyons, W., Fisher, T. C., and Conte, R. 1977. Origins of short latency auditory evoked potentials in man. In: J. E. Desmedt (ed.), Auditory Evoked Potentials in Man: Psychopharmacology Correlates of Evoked Potentials. S. Karger, Basel. Prog. Clin. Neurophysiol. 2:30–44.

Goldstein, M. H., Jr., and Kiang, N. Y. S. 1958. Synchrony of neural activity in electric responses evoked by transient acoustic stimuli. J. Acoust. Soc. Am. 30:107–114.

Hashimoto, I., Ishiyama, Y., and Tozuka, G. 1979. Bilaterally recorded brain stem auditory evoked responses: Their asymmetric abnormalities and lesions of the brain stem. Arch. Neurol. 36:161–167.

Hashimoto, I., Ishiyama, Y., Yoshimoto, T., and Nemoto, S. 1981. Brain stem auditory evoked potentials recorded directly from human brain stem and thalamus. Brain 104:841–859.

Hawes, M. D., and Greenberg, H. J. 1981. Slow brain stem responses (SN10) to tone pips in normally hearing newborns and adults. Audiology 20:113–122.

Hecox, K. 1975. Electrophysiological correlates of human auditory development. In: L. Cohen and P. Salapatek (eds.), Infant Perception: From Sensation to Cognition, Vol. II, pp. 151–191. Academic Press, New York.

Hecox, K., and Galambos, R. 1974. Brain stem auditory evoked responses in human infants and adults. Arch. Otolaryngol. 99:30–33.

Hoke, M. 1976. Cochlear microphonics in man and its probable importance in objective audiometry. In: R. J. Ruben, C. Elberling, and G. Salomon (eds.), Electrocochleography, pp. 41–54. University Park Press, Baltimore.

Javel, E., Mouney, D. F., McGee, J., and Walsh, E. J. 1982. Auditory brainstem responses during systemic infusion of lidocaine. Arch. Otolaryngol. 108:71–76.

Jerger, J., and Mauldin, L. 1978. Prediction of sensorineural hearing level from the brain stem evoked response. Arch. Otolaryngol. 104:456–461.

Jerger, J., Neely, J. G., and Jerger, S. 1980. Speech, impedance, and auditory brainstem response audiometry in brainstem tumors: Importance of a multiple test strategy. Arch. Otolaryngol. 106:218–223.

Jewett, D. L., Romano, M. N., and Williston, J. S. 1970. Human auditory evoked potentials: Possible brain stem components detected on the scalp. Science 167:1517–1518.

Jewett, D. L., and Williston, J. S. 1971. Auditory evoked far fields averaged from the scalp of humans. Brain 94:681–696.

Kevanishvili, Z. Sh. 1980. Sources of the human brainstem auditory evoked potential. Scand. Audiol. 9:75–82.

Kevanishvili, Z. Sh. 1981. Considerations of the sources of brainstem auditory evoked potential on the basis of bilateral asymmetry of its parameters. Scand. Audiol. 10: 197–202.

Kiang, N. Y. S. 1965. Discharge Patterns of Single Fibers in the Cat's Auditory Nerve. Research Monograph No. 35. MIT Press, Cambridge, Massachusetts.

Kiang, N. Y. S. 1975. Stimulus representation in the discharge patterns of auditory neurons. In: D. B. Tower (ed.), The Nervous System, Vol 3· Human Communication and Its Disorders, pp. 81–96. Raven Press, New York.

Kiang, N. Y. S., and Moxon, E. C. 1974. Tails of tuning curves of auditory nerve fibers. J. Acoust. Soc. Am. 55:620–630.

Kiang, N. Y. S., Moxon, E. C., and Kahn, A. R. 1976. The relationship of gross potentials recorded from the cochlea to single unit activity in the auditory nerve. In: R. J. Ruben, C. Elberling, and G. Salomon (eds.), Electrocochleography, pp. 95–115. University Park Press, Baltimore.

Klein, A. J., and Mills, J. H. 1981. Physiological and psychophysical measures from humans with temporary threshold shift. J. Acoust. Soc. Am. 70:1045–1053.

Klein, A. J., and Teas, D. C. 1978. Acoustically dependent latency shifts of BSER (wave V) in man. J. Acoust. Soc. Am. 63:1887–1895.

Laukli, E., and Mair, I. W. S. 1981. Early auditory-evoked responses: Filter effects. Audiology 20:300–312.

Lawrence, M., Nuttal, A. L., and Clapper, M. P. 1974. Electrical potentials and fluid boundaries within the organ of Corti. J. Acoust. Soc. Am. 55:122–138.

Lev, A., and Sohmer, H. 1972. Sources of averaged neural responses recorded in animal and human subjects during cochlear audiometry (electrocochleography). Arch. Ohr. Nas. Kehlk Heilk 201:79–90.

Lynn, G. E., Gilroy, J., Connelly Taylor, P., and Leiser, R. P. 1981. Binaural masking level differences in neurological disorders. Arch. Otolaryngol. 107:357–362.

Michalewski, H. J., Thompson, L. W., Patterson, J. V., Bowman, T. E., and Litzelman, D. 1980. Sex differences in the amplitudes and latencies of the human auditory brain stem potential. Electroenceph. Clin. Neurophysiol. 48:351–356.

Mitchell, C., and Clemis, J. D. 1977. Audiograms derived from the brain stem response. Laryngoscope 87:2016–2022.

Moffat, D. A. 1979. Transtympanic electrocochleography in Meniere's disease: Variation in the amplitude of the summating potential related to clinical status. Br. J. Audiol. 13:149–152.

Mogensen, F., and Kristensen, D. 1979. Auditory double click evoked potentials in multiple sclerosis. Acta Neurol. Scandinav. 59:96–107.

Mokotoff, B., Schulman-Galambos, C., and Galambos, R. 1977. Brain stem auditory evoked responses in children. Arch. Otolaryngol. 103:38–43.

and Jannetta, P. 1982. Neural generators of the brainstem auditory intial. In: Abstracts of the Fifth Midwinter Research Meeting. Association for Research in Otolaryngology. January, St. Petersburg, Florida.

Moller, A. R., Jannetta, P., and Moller, M. B. 1981. Neural generators of brainstem evoked potentials. Results of human intracranial recordings. Ann. Otol. 90:591–596.

Moller, A. R., Jannetta, P., and Moller, M. B. 1982. Intracranially recorded auditory nerve response in man: New interpretations of BSER. Arch. Otolaryngol. 108:77–82.

Moller, K., and Blegvad, B. 1976. Brain stem potentials in subjects with sensorineural hearing loss. Scand. Audiol. 5:115–127.

Moore, E. J. 1971. Human cochlear microphonics and auditory nerve action potentials from surface electrodes. Unpublished doctoral thesis, University of Wisconsin, Madison.

Naunton, R. F., and Zerlin, S. S. 1978. Electrocochleography: Behavioral threshold comparisons. In: R. F. Naunton and C. Fernandez (eds.), Evoked Electrical Activity in the Auditory Nervous System, pp. 221–236. Academic Press, New York.

Nishida, H., Kumagami, H., and Baba, M. 1981. Electrocochleographic study of patients with cerebral vascular lesions. Arch. Otolaryngol. 107:74–78.

Ochs, R., Markland, O. N., and DeMyer, W. E. 1979. Brainstem auditory evoked responses in leukodystrophies. Neurology 29:1089–1093.

Odenthal, D. W., and Eggermont, J. J. 1976. Electrocochleographic study of Meniere's disease and pontine angle neurinoma. In: R. J. Ruben, C. Elberling, and G. Salomon (eds.), Electrocochleography, pp. 331–352. University Park Press, Baltimore.

Ozdamar, O., and Dallos, P. 1976. Input-output functions of cochlear whole-nerve action potentials: Interpretation in terms of one population of neurons. J. Acoust. Soc. Am. 59:143–147.

Parker, D. J. 1981. Dependence of the auditory brainstem response on electrode location. Arch. Otolaryngol. 107:367–371.

Parker, D. J., and Thornton, A. R. D. 1978a. Cochlear traveling wave velocities calculated from the derived components of the cochlear nerve and brainstem evoked responses of the human auditory system. Scand. Audiol. 7:67–70.

Parker, D. J., and Thornton, A. R. D. 1978b. Frequency specific components of the cochlear nerve and brainstem evoked responses of the human auditory system. Scand. Audiol. 6:53–60.

Parker, D. J., and Thornton, A. R. D. 1978c. The validity of the cochlear nerve and brainstem evoked responses of the human auditory system. Scand. Audiol. 7:45–52.

Parving, A., Elberling, C., and Smith, T. 1981. Auditory electrophysiology: Findings in multiple sclerosis. Audiology 20:123–142.

Peck, M. A. 1979. Action potentials recorded from the promontory and ear canal simultaneously with induced middle ear liquids. Unpublished master's thesis, University of Arizona, Tucson.

Picton, T. W., Hillyard, S. A., Krausz, H. I., and Galambos, R. 1974. Human auditory evoked potentials. I. Evaluation of components. Electroenceph. Clin. Neurophysiol. 36:179–190.

Picton, T. W., Quellette, J., Hamel, G., and Smith, A. D. 1979. Brainstem evoked potentials to tone pips in notched noise. J. Otolaryngol. 8:289–314.

Picton, T. W., Woods, D. L., Baribeau-Braun, J., and Healey, T. M. G. 1977. Evoked potential audiometry. J. Otolaryngol. 6:90–119.

Portmann, M., and Aran, J.-M. 1972. Relations entre "pattern" électrocochléographique et pathologie rétro-labyrinthique. Acta Oto-laryng. 73:190–196.

Portmann, M., Cazals, Y., Negrevergne, M., and Aran, J. M. 1980. Transtympanic and surface recordings in the diagnosis of retrocochlear disorders. Acta Oto-laryng. 89:362–369.

Portmann, M., LeBert, G., and Aran, J.-M. 1967. Potentiels cochléaires obtenus chez l'homme en dehors toute intervention chirurgicale. Note préliminaire. Rev. Laryngol. Otol. Rhinol. (Bordeaux) 88:157–164.

Prasher, D. K., and Gibson, W. P. R. 1981. Phase reversal in brain stem responses: Its use in the detection of asymmetry in the auditory pathways. Audiology 20:313–324.

Pratt, H., and Sohmer, H. 1976. Intensity and rate functions of cochlear and brainstem evoked responses to click stimulation in man. Arch. Otorhinolaryngol. 212:85–92.

Reneau, J. P., and Hnatiow, G. Z. 1975. Evoked Response Audiometry: A Topical and Historical Review. University Park Press, Baltimore.

Roberts, J. L., Davis, H., Phon, G. L., Reichert, T. J., Sturtevant, B. S. N., and Marshall, R. E. 1982. Auditory brainstem responses in pre-term neonates: Maturation and follow-up. J. Pediatr. 101:257–263.

Robinson, K., and Rudge, P. 1977. The early components of the auditory evoked potential in multiple sclerosis. In: J. E. Desmedt (ed.), Auditory Evoked Potentials in Man: Psychopharmacology Correlates of Evoked Potentials, pp. 58–67. S. Karger, Basel.

Rose, D. E. Brainstem evoked responses in audiometry. In: B. Jazbi (ed.), Pediatric Otorhinolaryngology. Yearbook Medical Publishers, Chicago. In press.

Rosenhamer, H. J. 1977. Observations on electric brain-stem responses in retrocochlear hearing loss. Scand. Audiol. 6:179–196.

Rosenhamer, H. J., Lindstrom, B., and Lundborg, J. 1978. On the use of click-evoked electric brainstem responses in audiological diagnosis. I. The variability of the normal response. Scand. Audiol. 7:193–206.

Rosenhamer, H. J., Lindstrom, B., and Lundborg, J. 1980. On the use of click-evoked electric brainstem responses in audiological diagnosis. II. The influence of sex and age upon the normal response. Scand. Audiol. 9:93–100.

Rosenhamer, H. J., Lindstrom, B., and Lundborg, J. 1981a. On the use of click-evoked electric brainstem responses in audiological diagnosis. III. Latencies in cochlear hearing loss. Scand. Audiol. 10:3–11.

Rosenhamer, H. J., Lindstrom, B., and Lundborg, J. 1981b. On the use of click-evoked electric brainstem responses in audiological diagnosis. IV. Interaural latency differences (Wave V) in cochlear hearing loss. Scand. Audiol. 10:67–73.

Rowe, M. J. 1978. Normal variability of the brain stem auditory evoked response in young and old adult subjects. Electroenceph. Clin. Neurophysiol. 44:459–470.

Ruben, R. J., Elberling, C., and Salomon, G. (eds.), 1976. Electrocochleography. University Park Press, Baltimore.

Runge, C. A. 1980. Intracranial and surface recordings of the auditory brain stem response in the cat. Unpublished master's thesis, University of Arizona, Tucson.

Ryerson, S. G., and Beagley, H. A. 1981. Brainstem electric responses and electrocochleography: A comparison of threshold sensitivities in children. Br. J. Audiol. 15:41–48.

116   Short-Latency Auditory Evoked Potentials

Salamy, A., and McKean, C. M. 1976. Postnatal development of human brain-stem potentials during the first year of life. Electroenceph. Clin. Neurophysiol. 40:418–426.
Salamy, A., McKean, C. M., and Buda, F. B. 1975. Maturational changes in auditory transmission as reflected in human brain stem potentials. Brain Res. 96:361–366.
Salomon, G., and Elberling, C. 1971. Cochlear nerve potentials recorded from the ear canal in man. Acta Oto-laryng. 71:319–325.
Schulman-Galambos, C., and Galambos, R. 1975. Brainstem auditory evoked responses in premature infants. J. Speech Hear. Res. 18:456–465.
Selters, W. A., and Brackmann, D. E. 1977. Acoustic tumor detection with brain stem electric response audiometry. Arch. Otolaryngol. 103:181–187.
Selters, W. A., and Brackmann, D. E. 1979. Brainstem electric response audiometry in acoustic tumor detection. In: W. F. House and C. M. Leutje (eds.), Acoustic Tumors, Vol. I: Diagnosis, pp. 225–235. University Park Press, Baltimore.
Simmons, F. B., and Beatty, D. L. 1962. The significance of round window recorded cochlear potentials in hearing. Ann. Otol. 71:767–801.
Simmons, F. B., and Glattke, T. J. 1975. Electrocochleography. In: L. J. Bradford (ed.), Physiological Measures of the Audio-Vestibular System, pp. 147–175. Academic Press, New York.
Skinner, P., and Glattke, T. J. 1977. Electrophysiologic response audiometry: State of the art. J. Speech Hear. Dis. 42:179–198.
Sohmer, H., and Feinmesser, M. 1967. Cochlear action potentials recorded from the external ear in man. Ann. Otol. 76:427–435.
Sohmer, H., Kinarti, R., and Gafni, M. 1981. The latency of auditory nerve-brainstem responses in sensorineural hearing loss. Arch. Otorhinolaryngol. 230:189–199.
Sohmer, H., and Zuckerman, B. 1979. Recording of auditory nerve and brain-stem evoked responses with surface electrodes. In: H. A. Beagley (ed.), Auditory Investigation: The Scientific and Technological Basis, pp. 403–417. Clarendon Press, Oxford.
Spoendlin, H. 1973. The innervation of the cochlear receptor. In: A. R. Moller (ed.), Basic Mechanisms in Hearing. p. 185–234. Academic Press, New York.
Squires, N., Aine, C., Buchwald, J., Norman, R., and Galbraith, G. 1980. Auditory brain stem response abnormalities in severely and profoundly retarded adults. Electroenceph. Clin. Neurophysiol. 50:172–185.
Starr, A. 1976. Auditory brain-stem responses in brain death. Brain 99:543–554.
Starr, A., and Achor, J. 1975. Auditory brain stem responses in neurological disease. Arch. Neurol. 32:761–768.
Starr, A., Amlie, R. N., Martin, W. H., and Sanders, S. 1977. Development of auditory function in newborn infants revealed by auditory brainstem potentials. Pediatrics 60:831–839.
Starr, A., and Hamilton, A. E. 1976. Correlation between confirmed sites of neurological lesions and abnormalities of far-field auditory brainstem responses. Electroenceph. Clin. Neurophysiol. 41:595–608.
Stephens, S. D., and Thornton, A. R. D. 1976. Subjective and electrophysiologic tests in brain stem lesions. Arch. Otolaryngol. 102:608–613.
Stockard, J. E., Stockard, J. J., Westmoreland, B. F., and Corfits, J. L. 1979. Brainstem auditory evoked responses: Normal variation as a function of stimulus and subject characteristics. Arch. Neurol. 36:823–831.

Stockard, J. J., and Rossiter, V. S. 1977. Clinical and pathologic correlates of brain stem auditory response abnormalities. Neurology 27:316–325.

Stockard, J. J., Sharbrough, F. W., and Tinker, J. A. 1978. Effects of hypothermia on the human brainstem auditory response. Ann. Neurol. 3:368–370.

Stockard, J. J., Stockard, J. E., and Sharbrough, F. W. 1977. Detection and localization of occult lesions with brainstem auditory responses. Mayo Clinic Proc. 52:761–769.

Stockard, J. J., Stockard, J. E., and Sharbrough, F. W. 1978. Nonpathologic factors influencing brainstem auditory evoked potentials. Am. J. EEG Technol. 18:177–209.

Suzuki, T., Hirai, Y., and Horiuchi, K. 1977. Auditory brain stem responses to pure tone stimuli. Scand. Audiol. 6:51–56.

Tasaki, I., Davis, H., and Eldredge, D. H. 1954. Exploration of cochlear potentials in guinea pig with a microelectrode. J. Acoust. Soc. Am. 26:765–773.

Tasaki, I., Davis, H., and Legouix, J.-P. 1952. The space-time pattern of the cochlear microphonics (guinea pig) as recorded by differential electrodes. J. Acoust. Soc. Am. 24:502–519.

Teas, D. D., Eldredge, D. H., and Davis, H. 1962. Cochlear responses to acoustic transients: An interpretation of whole nerve action potentials. J. Acoust. Soc. Am. 34:1438–1459.

Terkildsen, K., and Osterhammel, P. 1981. The influence of reference electrode position on recordings of the auditory brainstem responses. Ear Hear. 2:9–19.

Terkildsen, K., Osterhammel, P., and Huis in't Veld, F. 1973. Electrocochleography with a far-field technique. Scand. Audiol. 2:141–148.

Terkildsen, K., Osterhammel, P., and Huis in't Veld, F. 1975. Far-field electrocochleography. Frequency specificity of the response. Scand. Audiol. 4:167–172.

Thornton, A. R. D. 1975. Bilaterally recorded early acoustic responses. Scand. Audiol. 4:173–181.

Thornton, A. R. D. 1976. Statistical properties of electrocochleographic responses and their use in clinical diagnosis. In: R. J. Ruben, C. Elberling, and G. Salomon (eds.), Electrocochleography, pp. 257–276. University Park Press, Baltimore.

Tobias, J. V., and Jeffress, L. A. 1962. Earphone response and onset time. J. Acoust. Soc. Am. 34:857–858.

von Bekesy, G. 1950. Experiments in Hearing. McGraw-Hill Book Company, New York.

Weiss, T. F., and Peake, W. T. 1972. Cochlear potential response at the round-window membrane of the cat: A reply to the comment of G. R. Price. J. Acoust. Soc. Am. 52:1729–1734.

Worthington, D. W., and Peters, J. F. 1980a. Electrophysiologic audiometry. Ann. Otol. Suppl. 74:59–62.

Worthington, D. W., and Peters, J. F. 1980b. Quantifiable hearing and no ABR: Paradox or error? Ear Hear. 1:281–285.

Yamada, O., Kodera, K., and Yagi, T. 1979. Cochlear processes affecting wave V latency of the auditory evoked brain stem response: A study of patients with sensory hearing loss. Scand. Audiol. 8:67–70.

Yamada, O., Toshiaki, Y., Yamane, H., and Suzuki, J. 1975. Clinical evaluation of the auditory evoked brain stem response. Auris. Nasis. Larynx (Tokyo) 2:97–105.

Yoshie, N. 1973. Diagnostic significance of the electrocochleogram in clinical audiometry. Audiology 12:504–539.

Yoshie, N. 1976. Electrocochleographic classification of sensorineural defects: Pathological pattern of the cochlear nerve compound action potential in man. In: R. J. Ruben, C. Elberling, and G. Salomon (eds.), Electrocochleography, pp. 353–386. University Park Press, Baltimore.

Yoshie, N., and Ohashi, T. 1969. Clinical use of cochlear nerve action potential responses in man for differential diagnosis of hearing losses. Acta Oto-laryng. Suppl. 252:71–87.

Yoshie, N., Ohashi, T., and Suzuki, T. 1967. Non surgical recording of auditory nerve action potentials in man. Laryngoscope 77:76–85.

Yoshie, N., and Yamaura, K. 1969. Cochlear microphonic responses to pure tones in man recorded by a non surgical method. Acta Oto-laryng. Suppl. 252:37–69.

Zerlin, S. S., and Naunton, R. F. 1976. Whole-nerve response to third octave audiometric clicks at moderate sensation level. In: R. F. Ruben, C. Elberling, and G. Salomon (eds.), Electrocochleography, pp. 199–206. University Park Press, Baltimore.

APPENDIX:
ILLUSTRATIVE CASES

INTRODUCTION

This section reviews test results and the subsequent clinical impressions for several individuals seen at the University of Arizona clinics over the past few years. Some of the results and impressions are straightforward and some were selected to illustrate unusual findings that may occur. The retrospective comments included with each case were developed at the time the materials for this book were assembled to stimulate the thinking of the reader regarding possible interpretive problems that will be encountered in a routine clinical practice.

All case reports should include: (1) relevant background information; (2) a description of the methods employed; (3) an objective statement of the results; (4) a comparison of those results with appropriate norms; and (5) a summary of impressions. The cases described in this appendix include the background information and, usually, a plot of the response latencies as a function of stimulus SPL so that the reader may quickly compare the measures obtained for an individual patient with our normal range. Our norms are based on young adult listeners with no hearing loss (10 dB or better from 250 through 8,000 Hz re: ANSI, 1969 standards) who were tested with unfiltered rarefaction clicks at a rate of 10 per second. Responses were recorded via electrodes placed at the vertex (noninverting), ipsilateral mastoid (inverting) and contralateral mastoid (common). The filter settings were 100 to 3,000 Hz, and two responses based on 1,000 samples were combined to produce representative responses. In clinical practice, we gather responses based on 1,000 samples and routinely repeat the data-gathering procedure to insure reliability for both high-intensity and near-threshold responses. The repetitions for the high-intensity responses are necessary to improve confidence in the interwave interval measurements, and the near-threshold replications help to confirm threshold estimates. We prefer to use a stimulus fixed in the rarefaction phase for ABR testing. Masking of the nontest ear is employed only when required (see Chapter 8).

All clinical test sessions begin with a control run using all normal computer, filter, and stimulus settings, but with the preamplifier inputs shorted. This permits an initial check of the amplification, stimulus generation, and computer system. Electrical artifacts that occur in this situation usually are related to radiation from the earphone leads to the cable between the preamplifier and computer mainframe. If uncorrected, they will continue to plague the examiner throughout the evaluation process. This is followed by sampling EEG activity from the patient electrodes without presenting a stimulus series, again to insure the absence of an artifact. If we are examining someone for the purpose of supplementing impressions based on behavioral hearing tests (e.g., infants, multiply handicapped children, and adults), we initiate the response recording with stimuli at 65 dB nHL (100 dB SPL) presented to the suspected "better" ear if that information is available. Beginning the sampling with stimuli of greater intensity often will arouse the patient from sleep. Threshold is sought by using a method of limits, descending in 20-dB steps from 60 dB nHL until no response is noted. The stimulus intensity is raised to the minimum SPL at which a response was observed, and a descending trial is initiated from that point using 10-dB steps. The minimum SPL at which a designated wave V makes its appearance on two of those descending trials is taken as the threshold. We do not test routinely below 15 dB nHL (50 dB SPL).

If no responses are observed for stimulation of the first ear at 65 dB nHL, we increase the stimulus SPL in 10-dB steps to the limits of the equipment, attempting to determine a threshold and as many suprathreshold points (in 10-dB steps) as possible. The common and inverting electrodes are then reversed at the preamplifier input and the other ear is evaluated.

We require audiometric information before applying the ABR procedures to cooperating adults for the purpose of neurologic assessment. Many patients who report no history of hearing loss and no communication difficulties have high-frequency loss that can obscure interpretation of the ABR findings. Where possible, such patients are evaluated by the determination of an ABR latency/intensity series that includes three or more measures of response latency at suprathreshold intensities (100, 110, 120, dB SPL). A significant hearing loss may preclude such determinations, and we discourage referrals for ABR procedures when the patient's hearing loss is known to be greater than 60 to 70 dB in the frequency region above 2,000 Hz.

If the primary purpose of the evaluation is to determine audiometric threshold and if the patient has been sedated, we are inclined to test at 20 or 30 clicks per second, rather than 10 per second, in order to optimize our data collection during the brief period of patient relaxation. The slower repetition rates are used for site-of-lesion studies because they improve the resolution of the earlier response components.

The usual nonpathologic causes of unreliable responses are inadequate electrode application and incomplete patient relaxation. The former can be detected by a check of the electrode impedance, and the latter can be controlled in cooperative patients with additional instruction. The ABR and associated EEG signals may be dominated by a post-auricular myogenic response in some individuals. We move the common and inverting electrodes to the medial surface of the earlobe in attempts to reduce the myogenic component.

Combined cochleographic and ABR studies are employed for site-of-lesion testing, especially for patients with history or symptoms that make them suspect for retrocochlear lesions. The special cochleographic procedures include placement of the noninverting (active) electrode in the external meatus and using the ipsilateral earlobe as the site for the inverting (reference) electrode. The forehead is used as a common electrode site. The preamplifier filter setting is changed to 10 to 3,000 Hz to allow a clear representation of the SP. The noise levels associated with the wider filter passband and the ear canal electrode are much greater than those encountered with routine ABR recording, and the "artifact" rejection option has to be defeated to obtain the records. The combined SP/AP response is obtained by collecting 1,000 or 2,000 samples using a rarefaction pulse, repeating that procedure using a condensation pulse, and by adding the two means together in the computer memory. This allows for inspection of the cochlear microphonic (and stimulus artifact) associated with each of the records before cancellation due to the computer summing process. In addition, the individual rarefaction record remains available for comparison with the ABR obtained with rarefaction clicks. We do not routinely test for "threshold" using cochleographic techniques, but use responses obtained at 100, 110, and 120 dB SPL to examine the SP and to provide indications of the latency of wave I when the latter is obscured in the ABR record.

Peak identification in the ABR record sometimes is difficult even though recordings are obtained in a technically competent manner. Wave

I may be elusive or obscured by electrical artifact. When selecting a point to represent the latency of wave I, it is wise to remember that the peak should be between about 1.2 and 1.5 msec for high-intensity stimuli, and never briefer than 1 msec (unless the computer initiates sampling after a delay of 0.2 to 0.5 msec).The blending of IV and V often makes specification of the latency of wave V difficult. The relative amplitudes of IV and V may be such that one can dominate the response and the other appear as only a small inflection point. Sometimes, recording the ABR with the inverting (reference) electrode on the contralateral mastoid or earlobe will help to separate the IV and V components, although changing the electrode site will also influence the apparent latency of the response.

The first six cases described in the following sections were cooperative individuals who were studied using our standard electrode placements and slow stimulus repetition rates. The twins described in Case 7 were studied with a hairline placement of the noninverting electrode and with stimuli at 30 per second.

CASE 1—ACOUSTIC NERVE TUMOR

This patient was 42 years of age and presented a unilateral sensorineural hearing loss as illustrated in Figure A.1. Speech discrimination scores were normal on the right and reduced on the left (66%). The speech

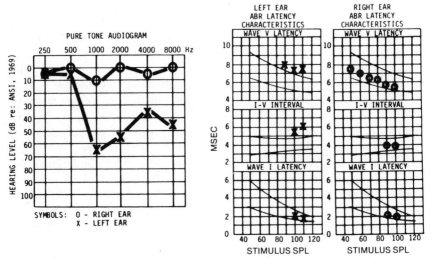

Figure A.1.   Audiometric and ABR latency results for Case 1. O = right ear; X = left ear.

discrimination score on the left also revealed a rollover effect for materials presented at high intensity. Tone decay screening was borderline for the left ear. Tympanometry results were normal and acoustic reflexes were present bilaterally without decay. Electronystagmography (ENG) and caloric results were normal.

The ABR results are illustrated in Figure A.2. Responses with normal morphology, latency, and threshold characteristics were noted for stimulation of the right ear. A designated wave V was observed for stimuli as low as 50 dB SPL (15 dB nHL). Wave I was noted at 90 and 100 dB SPL. The wave V portion of the response to high-intensity stimulation in the right ear appears as a blending of IV and V, and the specified latency was measured to the last distinct peak in the complex.

Responses for the left ear had a threshold of 90 dB SPL, or 55 dB nHL, in good approximation to the high-frequency portion of the audiogram. The latency of the near-threshold designated wave V is prolonged for stimuli at 90 dB SPL, but consistent with the hearing loss. Responses to stimuli at 100 and 110 dB SPL reveal a consistent pro-

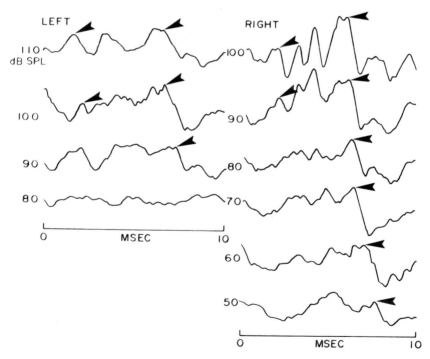

Figure A.2.   ABR tracings for Case 1. The arrows indicate the points chosen for wave I and wave V latency estimates.

longation of the *latency* of wave V and the *interval* between wave I and wave V.

At surgery, a 3- × 1.5-cm tumor was removed from the vestibular branch of the left auditory nerve.

Comment   In this case, the early ABR and audiometric results were helpful in dictating the eventual followup that permitted the diagnosis and successful removal of the tumor. The ABR findings in this instance reveal a probable I–V interval prolongation, and the ABR threshold elevation is consistent with the amount of high-frequency hearing loss on the left.

One interesting aspect of these results is that the responses obtained from the left ear to high-intensity stimuli lack clear definition, even though the near-threshold responses are similar to near-threshold responses obtained from the better ear. (The responses at 90 and 100 dB obtained for the left ear should be compared with the responses found for 50 to 70 dB stimuli on the right.) Many of our tumor patients reveal similar response characteristics, namely, fair response definition at low and moderate stimulus levels, and poor definition for high stimulus intensities.

CASE 2—ACOUSTIC NERVE TUMOR

This patient arrived at the clinic with a 6-month history of tinnitus in the left ear, unsteadiness, and headache. The audiogram, illustrated in Figure A.3, revealed normal thresholds through 2,000 Hz bilaterally and a slight threshold elevation in the very high frequencies. Speech discrimination was excellent bilaterally for materials presented at 45 dB HL. Tone decay screening was negative.

Tympanograms were normal, but no acoustic reflexes could be elicited for stimulation of the left ear. They were present on the left with stimulation of the right ear. No reflex decay was noted for reflexes due to right stimulation.

Electronystagmographic studies revealed a right-beating spontaneous nystagmus and hypoactive left vestibular response to caloric stimulation.

The ABR results are illustrated in Figure A.4. Responses obtained from the right ear were judged to be within normal limits in terms of latency and threshold characteristics. Wave V was not the most prominent response component at high stimulus intensities, and was designated as the small inflection on the negative slope of a IV/V complex. Wave I was present reliably at 90 and 110 dB SPL.

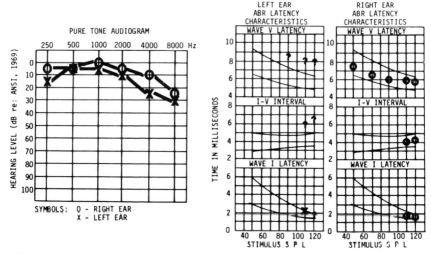

Figure A.3. Audiometric and ABR latency results for Case 2. O = right ear; X = left ear.

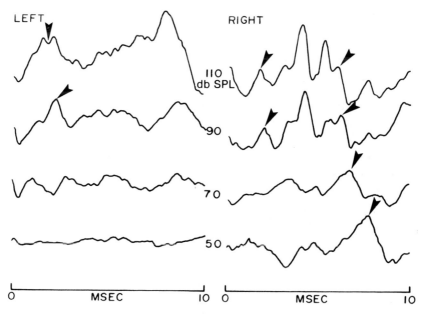

Figure A.4. ABR tracings for Case 2. The arrows indicate the points chosen for wave I and wave V latency estimates. The large delayed response on the left probably is due to a postauricular myogenic origin.

Responses obtained from stimulation of the left ear revealed gross waveform distortion. Wave I appeared to be the only reliable component present at high stimulus intensities. A large slow voltage fluctuation appeared with a prolonged latency at 110 and 120 dB SPL. (An example of the response to 110 dB is illustrated in the figure.)

Computerized axial tomography (CAT) with air contrast revealed a small space-occupying lesion contained within the left internal auditory meatus. At surgery, this was determined to be a mass arising from the auditory nerve and involving the facial nerve.

Comment   In this case, the acoustic reflex results prompted the ABR and ENG studies, and those prompted the air-contrast CAT studies that confirmed the presence of a tumor. There was no reliable indication of a wave V on the side of the lesion in this instance, and so this finding would not compare precisely with the ILD or I–V temporal measurements described in Chapter 8. The studies of patients with confirmed acoustic nerve tumors reviewed in Chapter 8 suggest that the absence of wave V is a common occurrence in those patients.

One must insure that the record has been obtained in a technically competent manner when this result is encountered. Convenient checks of the equipment can be made by (1) reversing the earphones and reevaluating both ears at a single suprathreshold intensity; and (2) retesting the better ear while recording from the electrodes used to measure responses from the poor ear. The second procedure will confirm the adequacy of the electrodes and other portions of the recording system.

CASE 3—SPACE-OCCUPYING LESION NOT INVOLVING THE AUDITORY NERVE

This case was a 29-year-old person who had a history of von Recklinghausen's disease. The patient had undergone prior surgery involving placement of a shunt for relief of mild hydrocephalus, and volunteered for audiological studies in order to assist us in a research project. The audiogram, illustrated in Figure A.5, indicated normal pure tone thresholds on the right and a slight sensorineural hearing loss in the mid- and high-frequency region on the left. Speech discrimination scores were reduced (86% right, 66% left) for materials presented at 40 dB above the speech reception threshold. There was no tone decay. Acoustic impedance results were normal and acoustic reflexes were present at normal threshold levels without reflex decay.

The ABR results generally were within normal limits for threshold and latency characteristics, although the I–V intervals were at the upper

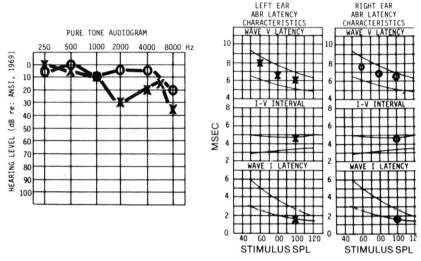

Figure A.5. Audiometric and ABR latency results for Case 3. *O* = right ear; *X* = left ear.

limit of the normal range. Responses to stimuli at 95 dB SPL are illustrated in Figure A.6.

Computerized axial tomography revealed an ovoid cystic area to the right of the midline and adjacent to or contiguous with the superior cerebellar cistern.

Comment   An interesting aspect of the ABR findings is the response waveform characteristic. The responses consisted of clear waves I, II, and III, and, on our initial reading, a designated wave V that was identified as such because of its amplitude and the following negative slope. Reexamination of the responses after consideration of the work of Parving, Elberling, and Smith (1981) suggests some possible alternative readings for the responses obtained from the right ear. The major peak, noted as V, was present with an absolute latency of 6.02 msec and a I–V interval of 4.8 msec. The small inflection point subsequent to the major peak was delayed by 0.5 msec (I–V interval of 5.3 msec), and the earlier small peak (noted as V?) provided an interval measurement of 4.1 msec. The small peak noted as V? was discounted as a probable wave V, even though it is the fifth peak in the response and the interval between it and wave I is closest to the mean for normal listeners. The major peak (V) was chosen because of its amplitude. Had the small inflection point to the right of the major peak been chosen, the interval measure and the absolute latency of the response would have

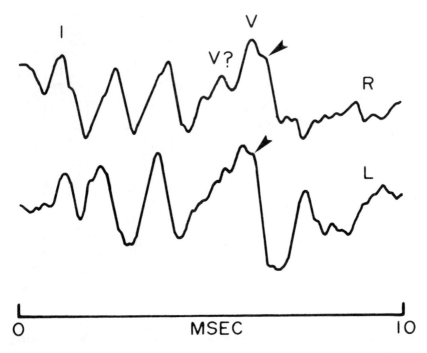

Figure A.6.   ABR tracings for right *(R)* and left *(L)* ear stimulation at 95 dB SPL in Case 3. The V?, V, and arrow in tracing *R* indicate possible choices for wave V in the case of the response of the right ear. The arrow in tracing *L* indicates the point chosen to represent wave V latency for the left ear.

been beyond two standard deviations from the normal mean values. By contrast, the small inflection point on the response taken from the left ear coincides with the designated V peak in the right ear response, and the entire response ensemble is more comfortably within normal limits. The relative heights of waves IV and V have been shown to be quite variable among subjects and stimulus conditions in the normal and clinical literature, and one often will encounter cases that present a number of decision alternatives regarding determination of the response peak latencies. Perhaps the most conservative route is to select a logical response component having the longest latency. If the resulting I–V interval measurement is within normal limits, the probability of making a false negative error would be low.

CASE 4—RISING AUDIOMETRIC CONFIGURATION

A 3-year-old was referred for hearing studies because of a severe delay of speech and language development. The medical history included recurring otitis media treated by pressure-equalization (PE) tubes at age 2 ½, but was otherwise not remarkable. The developmental history was marked by a general delay in gross motor skills and a failure to develop speech. Formal evaluation of speech and language development was difficult because the patient was unable to cooperate with the examiner.

An initial audiological evaluation using visual reinforcement techniques in sound field indicated that the speech awareness threshold was 40 dB HL. However, threshold responses to warbled tones between 250 and 4,000 Hz were found to range from 60 to 80 dB HL. The thresholds for tonal stimuli were much poorer than would have been predicted from the speech awareness threshold, and the reliability of the initial test results was judged to be poor.

This evaluation was followed by testing using ABR techniques with sedation. An ABR threshold of 25 dB nHL for click stimuli was noted for the left ear. No responses were obtained for stimulation of the right ear. Tympanometry results were consistent with a patent PE tube on the left. The tympanogram for the right ear revealed a negative middle ear pressure. Acoustic reflexes were absent for tonal stimuli between 500 and 4,000 Hz.

Repeated behavioral evaluations at the referring facility resulted in the determination of a reliable pure tone audiogram within approximately three months after the initial clinic visit. The audiogram for the left ear had a markedly rising characteristic, extending from 75 to 90 dB HL in the low-frequency region to 25 dB at 8 kHz. A profound loss was indicated for the right ear.

The patient returned to our facility at approximately age 4 at our request to determine if our initial ABR results could be repeated. By this time, the patient was able to cooperate with the examiner and sedation was not required for the ABR procedure. An audiogram obtained just prior to the second ABR study is illustrated in Figure A.7, along with the latency measures obtained from the second visit. The responses obtained for stimulation of the left ear are illustrated in Figure A.8. Clear, replicable responses were noted for stimulation of the left ear down to 25 dB nHL (60 dB SPL), in agreement with the results from the previous year. Additional behavioral testing at the time of the second ABR evaluation indicated that thresholds for warbled high-frequency tonal stimuli (8,000 to 16,000 Hz) were identical to those of young adult listeners tested under the same conditions.

Comment The initial pure tone and speech awareness threshold discrepancies can be explained on the basis of the patient's high-frequency hearing sensitivity. The excellent ABR results correspond well with the patient's threshold at 8,000 Hz on the conventional audiogram

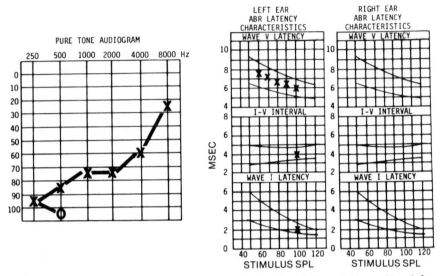

Figure A.7.   Audiometric and ABR latency results for Case 4. *O* = right ear; *X* = left ear.

and they provide no hint as to the extent of hearing loss through the mid- and low-frequency regions. Given that the high-frequency hearing sensitivity was normal, the amount of low-frequency hearing loss in this case was unusually large. The pure tone audiogram probably reflects a mixed loss with both conductive and sensorineural components. These findings demonstrate that ABR threshold findings must be interpreted only in the context of high-frequency hearing sensitivity when clicks are used as the eliciting stimulus.

CASE 5—SUDDEN HEARING LOSS

This patient was 48 years of age when seen for ABR studies. Approximately two months prior to the clinic visit, the patient had undergone coronary bypass surgery. A sudden hearing loss in the right ear was noted 18 days after surgery. A similar loss in the left ear was noted about two weeks later. The audiometric results are illustrated in Figure A.9. The pure tone results identified as "pre" were obtained about 10 years prior to the surgery. Those labelled "post" were obtained at the time of the ABR evaluation. Speech discrimination scores were below 10% bilaterally. Acoustic reflexes were present for 500 Hz bilaterally at reduced sensation levels. They were absent for higher frequencies. The patient was able to follow conversational speech with speechreading cues very

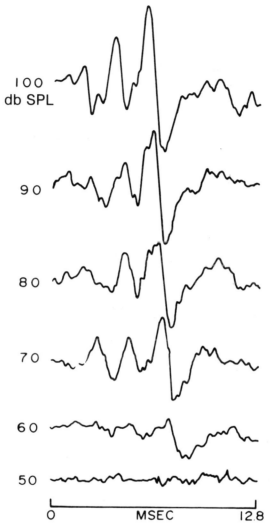

Figure A.8.   ABR tracings for stimulation of the left ear of Case 4. No responses were obtained for stimulation of the right ear.

competently, and the referral for ABR studies was made to help rule out significant functional hearing loss.

The ABR results are illustrated in Figure A.10. Responses for the left ear reveal a designated wave V with a prolonged latency and threshold of approximately 100 dB SPL (65 dB nHL). Responses for the right ear were characterized by poor definition and minimal changes of latency with changes in stimulus intensity.

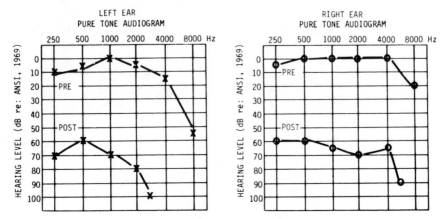

Figure A.9.   Audiometric results for Case 5.

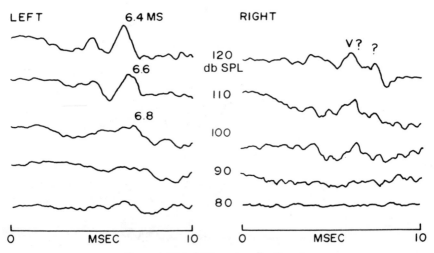

Figure A.10.   ABR tracings for Case 5.

Comment   While it is our practice to discourage referrals for click-evoked ABR studies if the patient's hearing loss exceeds 60 dB HL at 4,000 Hz and above, this patient was evaluated because of the physician's concern for possible significant functional hearing loss. The response characteristics correspond with the presence of a bilateral high-frequency hearing loss that is greater than that indicated on the "pre" audiograms, but they reflect the uncertainty of estimating thresholds reviewed in Chapter 8. Specifically, we expected to find responses that followed a pattern just opposite to that which was encountered. Minimal responses were anticipated for both ears, but we expected clearer responses from the right ear than from the left because of the better hearing at 4,000 Hz on the right.

These responses also illustrate the problems associated with attempting to estimate site of lesion based on ABR measures in the presence of significant high-frequency hearing loss. The responses at 120 dB SPL (85 dB nHL) are prolonged and do not provide a clear wave I. Interwave interval measurements cannot be obtained and the test results are not definitive.

CASE 6—UNILATERAL SUDDEN HEARING LOSS

This case involves a 58-year-old who presented a lengthy history of noise exposure and an accompanying bilateral high-frequency sensorineural hearing loss. Two and a half months prior to the visit to our clinic, the patient experienced a sudden decrease in hearing on the left. This was accompanied by constant tinnitus. On the day of the clinic visit, the audiogram revealed a bilateral sensorineural hearing loss, as illustrated in Figure A.11. Speech discrimination scores were 100% on the right and 56% on the left for materials presented at 35 dB above the speech reception threshold. There was reduced tolerance for speech on the left. There was no significant tone decay. Tympanometry studies were normal and acoustic reflexes were present without decay at reduced sensation levels for stimuli presented to the left ear.

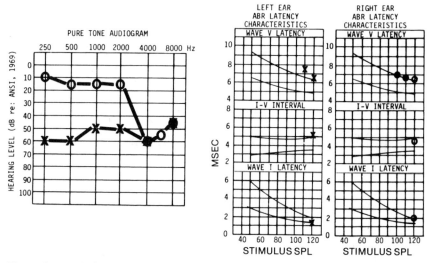

Figure A.11.   Audiometric and ABR latency results for Case 6. O = right ear; X = left ear.

The whole nerve AP responses obtained for stimulation at 120 dB SPL are illustrated in Figure A.12. The ABR resulting from stimulation of the right ear had fair definition of wave V, but there was no clear wave I. The absolute latency of wave V was slightly prolonged for all intensities at which it could be recorded. However, the AP response also revealed a prolonged latency, and the AP-V interval was within normal limits at 120 dB SPL.

Responses obtained from the left ear had poorer definition, a prolonged wave V, an increase in the AP-V interval, and an abnormal AP response waveform. The AP response was multipeaked, with an initial peak latency of 1.2 msec. This very brief latency was unexpected. The multipeaked finding was similar to that often found with Ménière's patients (cf. Chapter 6).

The ultimate diagnosis in this case was that the sudden increase in hearing loss on the left was due to cochlear disorder, although the patient's symptoms were not entirely suggestive of a classic Ménière's syndrome.

CASE 7—PREMATURE TWINS

Twins born at a conceptional age of 32 weeks were referred to hearing evaluation at the time they were dismissed from the intensive-care nursery (36 weeks). One individual had weighed 1.3 kg at birth and the larger twin weighed 1.7 kg at birth. Both experienced respiratory distress and

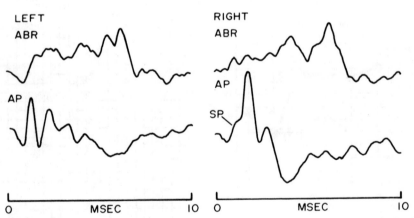

Figure A.12.   ABR and cochleography results for Case 6. The responses were obtained at 120 dB SPL. The AP response polarity has been plotted with the *negative peaks upward* to permit comparison with the ABR tracings. The AP/SP response on the right reveals a normal waveform. The response on the left is multipeaked, and has a very brief latency (1.2 msec).

an episode of jaundice. Both had received a three-day course of anti-biotics.

During behavioral observation, the smaller twin *(A)* failed to startle to tones or speech in the range of 90 to 100 dB HL, while the larger twin *(B)* had responses appropriate for age. The ABR results are illustrated in Figure A.13. No reliable responses were obtained for twin *A*, but responses were obtained from twin *B* at 60 dB SPL (about 25 dB nHL for adults).

They were reevaluated at a conceptional age of 45 weeks. Both were found to startle to speech at 65 dB HL and to alert to speech and warbled tones at levels consistent with their age. ABR results revealed responses at 60 dB SPL in both cases. Continuing followup during the first year of life has not indicated any suggestion of hearing loss.

Comment The initial findings from twin *A*, in the absence of significant neurological disorder, were suggestive of a hearing loss, but normal responses were obtained nine weeks later. In this case, the ABR was not useful in the prediction of permanent hearing impairment and we can only speculate about the absence of the responses in the smaller twin. That individual may have been experiencing a reversible (conductive) hearing loss or may have been exhibiting a maturational delay that

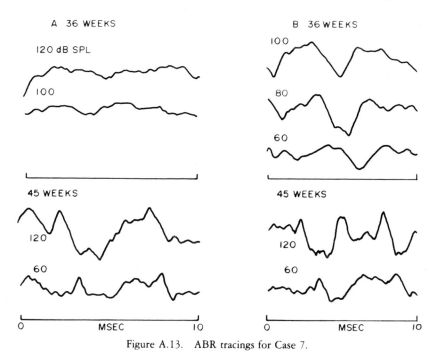

Figure A.13. ABR tracings for Case 7.

was reflected in the ABR. Based on similar experiences with other infants tested before 40 weeks' conceptional age and on the reports appearing more recently in the literature, we have elected to encourage referrals for ABR evaluations with infants after they reach 48 weeks' conceptional age. This is easily accommodated during the child's visit to the well-baby clinic and the ABR findings can be bolstered with more refined audiological measures as well as impressions of the parents, pediatric neurologists, and pediatricians.

SUMMARY

The examples selected for this appendix include a range of problems that may be encountered in a routine clinical practice. Significant hearing loss confined to the low-frequency region will be missed by ABR measures based on click stimuli. The response threshold for clicks should be a good indicator of high-frequency hearing sensitivity, but one will sometimes not be able to determine which ear is better in cases of bilateral hearing loss. This has important limiting implications for any attempt to prescribe hearing aids based on the results of ABR measurements.

Occasionally, identification of the appropriate response component for purposes of latency measurement may be difficult, and misidentification may occur if the "largest" response wave is always taken as wave V. One may also find responses with increased latencies that are difficult to interpret in terms of hearing loss or site of lesion.

As has been implied throughout this book, the short-latency evoked potentials offer great *sensitivity* to a variety of disorders. Our ability to interpret the information provided by the response characteristics is limited by that sensitivity in a very real sense. Neurologic problems (e.g., of multiply handicapped persons) can result in a failure of the response to appear even though hearing sensitivity for pure tones is normal. Hearing loss can obscure the responses to preclude neurologic interpretation. As with all other specialized tests, the results of the cochleography and ABR procedures should not be interpreted in isolation, and great caution would be exercised when making inferences based upon the responses. Cautious interpretation not only is in the best interests of the patient, but also of the clinical and scientific community at large.

INDEX